The Professional Lifespan: From Residency to Retirement

Editors

JINNY S. HA
STEPHEN C. YANG

THORACIC SURGERY CLINICS

www.thoracic.theclinics.com

Consulting Editor
VIRGINIA R. LITLE

February 2024 • Volume 34 • Number 1

ELSEVIER

1600 John F. Kennedy Boulevard • Suite 1800 • Philadelphia, Pennsylvania, 19103-2899

http://www.thoracic.theclinics.com

THORACIC SURGERY CLINICS Volume 34, Number 1
February 2024 ISSN 1547-4127, ISBN-13: 978-0-443-13023-6

Editor: John Vassallo (j.vassallo@elsevier.com)
Developmental Editor: Isha Singh

Thoracic Surgery Clinics (ISSN 1547-4127) is published quarterly by Elsevier Inc., 360 Park Avenue South, New York, NY 10010-1710. Months of publication are February, May, August, and November. Business and editorial offices: 1600 John F. Kennedy Boulevard, Suite 1800, Philadelphia, PA 19103-2899. Periodicals postage paid at New York, NY, and additional mailing offices. Subscription prices are $434.00 per year (US individuals), $100.00 per year (US students), $487.00 per year (Canadian individuals), $100.00 per year (Canadian students), $225.00 per year (international students), $524.00 per year (international individuals). For institutional access pricing please contact Customer Service via the contact information below Foreign air speed delivery is included in all Clinics' subscription prices. All prices are subject to change without notice. **POSTMASTER:** Send address changes to Thoracic Surgery Clinics, Elsevier Health Sciences Division, Subscription Customer Service, 3251 Riverport Lane, Maryland Heights, MO 63043. **Customer Service (orders, claims, online, change of address): Telephone: 1-800-654-2452 (U.S. and Canada); 314-447-8871 (outside U.S. and Canada). Fax: 314-447-8029. E-mail: journalscustomerservice-usa@elsevier.com (for print support); journalsonlinesupport-usa@elsevier.com (for online support).**

Reprints. For copies of 100 or more, of articles in this publication, please contact Commercial Rights Department, Elsevier Inc., 360 Park Avenue South, New York, NY 10010-1710. Tel: 212-633-3874; Fax: 212-633-3820; E-mail: reprints@elsevier.com.

Thoracic Surgery Clinics is covered in *MEDLINE/PubMed (Index Medicus), EMBASE/Excerpta Medica, Science Citation Index Expanded (SciSearch®), Journal Citation Reports/Science Edition,* and *Current Contents®/Clinical Medicine.*

Contributors

CONSULTING EDITOR

VIRGINIA R. LITLE, MD
Chief of Thoracic Surgery, Steward Medical
Group Thoracic Surgery, Brighton,
Massachusetts, USA

EDITOR

JINNY S. HA, MD, MHS
Assistant Professor of Thoracic Surgery, The
Johns Hopkins Medical Institutions, Division of
Thoracic Surgery, Department of Surgery,
Baltimore, Maryland

STEPHEN C. YANG, MD, FACS, MAMSE
The Arthur B. and Patricia B. Modell Endowed
Chair of Thoracic Surgery, Vice Chair for

Professional Development, Professor of
Surgery and Oncology, The Johns Hopkins
Medical Institutions, Division of Thoracic
Surgery, Department of Surgery, Baltimore,
Maryland

AUTHORS

WILLIAM A. BAUMGARTNER, MD
Inaugural Chair, The Academy at Johns
Hopkins, East Baltimore Campus, Emeritus
Professor, Surgery, Distinguished University
Service Professor, Baltimore, Maryland

FAIZ Y. BHORA, MD, FACS
Professor and Regional Chairman of Surgery,
Chief of Thoracic Surgery, Department of
Surgery, Hackensack Meridian School of
Medicine, Hackensack Meridian Health (HMH)
Network, Edison, New Jersey

MARKO T. BOSKOVSKI, MD, MHS, MPH
Assistant Professor of Surgery, Division of
Adult Cardiothoracic Surgery, Department of
Surgery, University of California, San
Francisco, San Francisco VA Medical Center,
San Francisco, California

ROBERT JAMES CERFOLIO, MD, MBA
Professor of Cardiothoracic Surgery at NYU,
Director of Quality and Lung Cancer Center,
Department of Cardiothoracic Surgery, NYU
Langone, New York, New York

ANDREW C. CHANG, MD
John Alexander Distinguished Professor,
Head of the Section of Thoracic Surgery,
University of Michigan, Ann Arbor,
Michigan

KRISTINE CHIN, BS
Lewis Katz School of Medicine at Temple
University, Philadelphia, Pennsylvania

MELANIE A. EDWARDS, MD
Site Medical Director, Thoracic Surgery,
Thoracic Surgeon, Cardiovascular and
Thoracic Surgery, Trinity Medical Group
Ann Arbor, Ypsilanti, Michigan

CHERIE P. ERKMEN, MD
Professor, Thoracic Surgery, Program Director,
ACGME Thoracic Surgery Fellowship, Temple
University Health Systems, Professor, Center
for Asian Health, Department of Thoracic
Medicine and Surgery, Lewis Katz School of
Medicine at Temple University, Philadelphia,
Pennsylvania

KIRSTEN A. FREEMAN, MD
Assistant Professor Cardiovascular Surgery, Department of Surgery, Division of Cardiovascular Surgery, University of Florida, Gainesville, Florida

BARBARA HAMILTON, MD
Clinical Assistant Professor, Department of Cardiac Surgery, Section of Adult Cardiac Surgery, University of Michigan Medical Center, Ann Arbor, Michigan

JASON J. HAN, MD
Division of Cardiovascular Surgery, Department of Surgery, University of Pennsylvania, Philadelphia, Pennsylvania

TARYNE A. IMAI, MD, MEHP
Associate Professor of Surgery, Director, Thoracic Surgery, Department of Surgery, Queen's University Health System, University of Hawaii, Honolulu, Hawaii

SARAH KHALIL, MD
Department of General Surgery, Western Michigan University, Homer Stryker MD School of Medicine, Kalamazoo, Michigan

RACHEL KIM, MD
Chief Resident, Cardiothoracic Surgery, The Ohio State University Wexner Medical Center, Columbus, Ohio

RUSSELL SETH MARTINS, MD
Postdoctoral Research Fellow, Division of Thoracic Surgery, Department of Surgery, Hackensack Meridian School of Medicine, Hackensack Meridian Health (HMH) Network, Edison, New Jersey

NAHUSH A. MOKADAM, MD
Professor, Director, Division of Cardiac Surgery, G.S. Kakos, MD and T.E. Williams, Jr., MD, PhD Endowed Professor in Cardiac Surgery, Associate Director, Surgical Services, Heart and Vascular Center, The Ohio State University Wexner Medical Center, Columbus, Ohio

KEITH S. NAUNHEIM, MD
The Vallee and Melba Willman Professor of Surgery, Chief of Thoracic Surgery, St Louis University School of Medicine

TOM C. NGUYEN, MD
Chief of Cardiothoracic Surgery, Division of Adult Cardiothoracic Surgery, San Francisco, California

ANNA OLDS, MD
Division of Cardiac Surgery, Department of Surgery, Keck School of Medicine of USC, University of Southern California, Los Angeles, California

HIMANSHU J. PATEL, MD
Joe D. Morris Collegiate Professor, Section Head, Adult Cardiac Surgery, Department of Cardiac Surgery, Executive Director, Cardiovascular Network of West Michigan, University of Michigan Medical Center, Ann Arbor, Michigan

JENNIFER L. PERRI, MD, MBA
Clinical Associate, Division of Cardiovascular and Thoracic Surgery, Duke University Medical Center, Durham, North Carolina

STEFANIE L. PETERS, MPA, LMSW, FACHE
Department of Cardiac Surgery, Frankel Cardiovascular Center, University of Michigan Medical Center, Ann Arbor, Michigan

JOSEPH J. PLATZ, MD
Assistant Professor of Surgery, St Louis University School of Medicine, St Louis, Missouri

KOSTANTINOS POULIKIDIS, MD, FACS
Assistant Professor, Division of Thoracic Surgery, Department of Surgery, Hackensack Meridian School of Medicine, Hackensack Meridian Health (HMH) Network, Edison, New Jersey

OURANIA PREVENTZA, MD, MBA, FACS
Professor of Surgery, Division of Cardiothoracic Surgery, Michael E. DeBakey Department of Surgery, Baylor College of Medicine, Academic Professional Staff, Department of Cardiovascular Surgery, The Texas Heart Institute, Attending Cardiovascular Surgeon, Department of Cardiovascular Surgery, St. Luke's Health— Baylor St Luke's Medical Center, Houston, Texas; Professor of Surgery, Division of Cardiothoracic Surgery, University of Virginia,

Co-Director of Cardiovascular Service Line
University of Virginia Health, Charlottesville,
Virginia

ELAINE E. TSENG, MD
Professor of Surgery, Division of Adult
Cardiothoracic Surgery, Department of
Surgery, University of California, San
Francisco, San Francisco VA Medical Center,
San Francisco, California

FATIMA G. WILDER, MD, MSc
Division of Thoracic Surgery, Department of
Surgery, Brigham and Women's Hospital,
Boston, Massachusetts

AMELIA W. WONG, DO
General Surgery Resident, Department
of Surgery, Queen's University Health
System, University of Hawaii, Honolulu,
Hawaii

Contents

> Quality mentorship is essential for a successful career in cardiothoracic surgery. From the premedical phase to the position of senior faculty, there are many benefits to having mentors who can provide insight, promote career advancement and facilitate professional opportunities. It is important to distinguish between a mentor and sponsor in seeking this career guidance because both are beneficial but serve different purposes. By being clear about one's professional goals, the mentor–mentee relationship can be optimized and lead to a fulfilling and productive career.

> Advanced training in cardiothoracic surgery has become more prevalent in the setting of increased complexity of interventions. Minimally invasive techniques, transcatheter and endovascular interventions, and rapid growth in mechanical circulatory support and transplant have led approximately 40% of trainees to pursue additional training. Available data suggest trainees seek additional training for 3 main reasons: gain an additional skillset, improve candidacy for a job, and/or increase proficiency in basic areas. This review provides an analysis of existing literature, categorized by specialty (cardiac, thoracic, and congenital) to determine areas where additional training is of benefit.

> It is a daunting task to find the "right" first job. However, the foundation of the search is similar to that of the interview and match process for residency and fellowship. Does the job opportunity have the makeup of clinical and research opportunities, case mix, support and culture that will set the trainee up to fulfill his or her early career goals? Does the position seem like a good fit? The variation occurs with (1) the mystery behind it—there are scarce resources available on the topic, and (2) the logistics: where and when to look; the interview process.

> New attending surgeons should consider hiring a Certified Financial Planner with experience in the surgical profession while also utilizing accessible resources to improve their financial literacy. They should acquire adequate life and disability insurance, devise debt-repayment strategies, and plan for retirement by contributing to tax-advantaged accounts and diversifying investments. New attending surgeons

should also be cognizant of the financial implications of important personal life events, such as marriage and childbirth. Having a financial team is important, and this may consist of a financial advisor and surgeon mentors.

There are several transitions that must be made to define your new role as an attending surgeon. Establishing these transitions can be difficult but trying to promote yourself while undergoing these awkward transitions can be taxing but nevertheless crucial. Whether you are in private practice trying to obtain referrals to build your practice or in an academic setting where you are trying to find your niche, promoting yourself along the way is imperative for your future growth. There are 3 core transitions in the first 5 years: (1) clinical, (2) professional, and (3) personal.

Cardiothoracic training continues to evolve and is a completely different teaching environment than prior. Cardiothoracic surgical educators are tasked to ensure that all levels of learners are appropriately trained. To be an effective surgical educator, one must expand their skills beyond being content experts but also acquire knowledge of educational theory and formal training in how to teach effectively. Furthermore, applying a scholarly approach and engaging in scholarship differentiate a cardiothoracic surgical educator from a teacher. Therefore, the surgical educator academic track is different from a surgical scientist track in terms of skills, work performed, documentation, and promotion requirements.

The academic promotion process in thoracic surgery can appear nebulous to many young surgeons. However, at most institutions, clear promotion criteria exist for specific academic tracks, and they are based on factors such as clinical excellence, research/investigation, funding, education/teaching, service, health policy, diversity, equity, and inclusion (DEI), ethics, quality and safety, and health care delivery. A thorough understanding of the promotion process is the key to successful advancement in academia.

In this article, we ask the reader to fully vet why they want to lead and who they want to lead. We then describe the different leaderships styles needed to effectively lead and deliver executive outcomes. We discuss the novel concept of different coachability styles and explain how an effective leader must understand when to apply one leadership style over another and which person of team will respond better to style over the others. The novel metric called the EQI—the efficiency quality index—by definition prevents this problem and is described and discussed.

Well-being is a quality of positive physical, mental, social, and environmental experiences. Well-being enables thoracic surgeons to achieve their full potential across personal and work domains. Evidence-based guidelines to promote individual well-being include (1) progress toward a goal; (2) actions commensurate with experience, interest, mission; (3) interconnectivity with others; (4) social relatedness of the work one does; (5) safety; and (6) autonomy. Successful pursuit of well-being includes the development of individual skills of mindfulness, resilience, and connection with others. However, well-being among individuals cannot be achieved without support of workplace leaders and durable institutional infrastructure.

Integrating Advocacy into Your Practice

Keith S. Naunheim and Joseph J. Platz

In the last 60 years, health care has evolved due to many trends including the introduction of third-party payers, a progressively aging society, advancing technology, emerging recognition of social issues of race/gender/poverty, the relative decline in the physician workforce, rising health care costs, ongoing consolidation of health care entities, and the corporatization of health care delivery. This has led to problems in health care delivery with respect to cost, quality, and access. Many medical leaders feel it is now the duty of the physician to go beyond the classic patient-doctor clinical responsibility and work to advocate for their patients and society regarding economic, financial, educational, and social issues.

The Mid-Career Crisis: Moving on to Your Next Job or Staying Comfortable

Ourania Preventza

The mid-career in a surgeon's life is not well defined in the literature. I define the mid-career as having two phases: the early phase, which is approximately 10 to 15 years in practice, and the later phase, which is at 15 to 25 years. However, these ranges are not the same for all; what matters is experience, exposure, repetition, and judgment, which come with time and commitment. During the mid-career, a surgeon becomes more confident in mastering techniques and teaching the next generation. If one's next job is a leadership position, one must realize that leadership is not about oneself but about elevating others.

Diversity in the Cardiothoracic Surgery Workforce: What I Can Do

Melanie A. Edwards

Within the cardiothoracic surgery workforce, there are significant gaps in the numbers of women and underrepresented in medicine minorities, but some progress has been made in gender diversity at the resident level. Individual surgeons play an important role in combatting discrimination and harassment, while also promoting women and minorities through mentorship and sponsorship. More importantly, a multifaceted and structured approach is needed to increase diversity at the institutional level with strategies to create a culture of inclusion, working to retain underrepresented minority and female surgeons, and eliminating bias in the recruitment process.

Surgical Citizenship: Engagement in Surgical Organizations

Himanshu J. Patel, Stefanie L. Peters, Barbara Hamilton, and Andrew C. Chang

As leaders, cardiothoracic surgeons must learn about and undergo transitions during the stages of a successful career. The authors discuss the process of transitions and the roles of networks to support professional transitions. The role of engagement in surgical organizations to create these networks and help support professional transitions is also explored. Finally, the authors describe how our engagement in surgical organizations can successfully impact our specialty of cardiothoracic surgery.

Retiring from any occupation is difficult, especially one that you love. The majority of cardiothoracic surgeons love what they do every day. It has been said that if you choose a job you love, you never have to work another day in your life. Once a date is determined, preparation, particularly financial, is paramount for a successful outcome. Thoughtful decisions need to be made regarding health benefits and retirement plans [401(k)/403(b)]. Transitions to retirement programs have been instituted in several schools of medicine. Establishing an academy for retired faculty can be an enriching experience for the members and a resource for the institution.

THORACIC SURGERY CLINICS

SERIES OF RELATED INTEREST

Advances in Surgery
http://www.advancessurgery.com/

Surgical Clinics
http://www.surgical.theclinics.com/

Surgical Oncology Clinics
https://www.surgonc.theclinics.com/

THE CLINICS ARE AVAILABLE ONLINE!
Access your subscription at:
www.theclinics.com

THORACIC SURGERY CLINICS

Foreword

From Residency to Retirement—Stop and Smell the Flowers

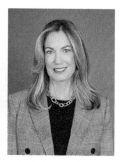

Virginia R. Litle, MD
Consulting Editor

First, I wish to thank Dr Stephen Yang for suggesting the topic of this issue of *Thoracic Surgery Clinics* entitled "From Residency to Retirement" and for engaging his Johns Hopkins' colleague Dr Jinny Ha to co-guest edit. With our professional lives continuing to evolve with more complex technical approaches and with our personal lives often taking a backseat to our jobs, we were due for a current handbook on how to proceed out the starting gate after a long and dedicated (and arduous many would justly say) educational prologue. Although a few contributions in this issue are oriented primarily to academic surgeons, many are relevant to all. Understanding personal finances as outlined by Drs Martins, Poulikidis, and Bhora is crucial to secure a comfortable lifestyle—when you retire! And Dr Baumgartner expands on the financial components of retirement but more importantly reminds us that there is life—and joy—after retirement.

With the implementation of work-hour limitations for trainees and with the constant advances in interventional therapies, Drs Perri and Nguyen address the topic of Advanced Fellowships and whether they are necessary to be successful. The bottom line is the authors suggest they are, but another option when feasible is to identify a CT residency earlier that would offer a higher volume of the technology that excites you, so you're prepared when looking for that first job, or if you're not fortunate to have matched at such a place, then taking a job where you have the mentorship to learn on the job. We read from Drs Wilder's and Han's piece about "Finding the Right Mentor." This topic is relevant to all new graduates, as we can fumble clinically or academically if we try to go it alone and that hurts not only our patients but also ourselves. The authors' key message is the value of a "mosaic mentorship" as one size does not fit all. Drs Kim and Mokadam expand on the mentor topic when summarizing the "right" first job. Do not be shy about asking someone (besides an attorney) to review your contract if it is one of the nonacademic formulaic ones full of legal lingo. If it is an academic position, don't hesitate to ask for start-up money for laboratory research or a database coordinator and/or statistician. Ask the mentor to review your offer!

One of the more unique topics covered in this issue is the value of "Integrating Advocacy into Your Practice," as authored by Dr Naunheim, who I deem a role model for advocacy, and I don't mean on the financial reimbursement side but on the patient and societal side. He reminds us that medicine selects altruistic individuals, so let's walk the talk.

Another topic relevant to all readers is "Implementation of Well-Being" as addressed by one of our specialty authorities, Dr Erkmen, and her national colleagues. The bottom line is a walk (or

Thorac Surg Clin 34 (2024) xiii–xiv
https://doi.org/10.1016/j.thorsurg.2023.09.004
1547-4127/24/© 2023 Published by Elsevier Inc.

thoracic.theclinics.com

run!) down this career highway can be exhilarating, but if we hit mental and physical obstacles, it won't matter if we have start-up money and incredible skill sets. We must have a holistic approach and recognize the value of mindfulness, resilience, and connection.

Thank you to Drs Ha and Yang and to all the contributors of this issue, a guidebook for our constantly challenging and intellectually stimulating professional road. The field of cardiothoracic surgery selects out folks who thrive on having a daily sense of purpose, a set of goals, and a desire to innovate and evolve. Many of us follow the words of Ralph Waldo Emerson: "Do not follow where the path may lead. Go instead where there is no path and leave a trail." We can be on the path as summarized in these articles, and we can contribute to advances in our field; however, if we don't care for ourselves, we will hit a dead end.

Virginia R. Litle, MD
St. Elizabeth's Medical Center
736 Cambridge Street
Cambridge, MA 02135, USA

E-mail address:
Vlitle@gmail.com

Twitter: @vlitlemd (V.R. Litle)

Preface

A Roadmap to Surgical Success: Your Path to a Rewarding Career

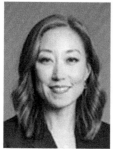

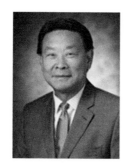

Jinny S. Ha, MD, MHS   Stephen C. Yang, MD, FACS, MAMSE

Editors

Embarking on a career in cardiothoracic surgery is an odyssey defined by unwavering commitment to treating cardiothoracic diseases and propelling the field forward. "The Professional Lifespan: From Residency to Retirement" is a scholarly exploration that intricately navigates this journey.

A career in cardiothoracic surgery is a complex tapestry, elaborately woven from the fabric of rigorous training, clinical and technical mastery, and steadfast dedication to patient care. This issue dissects the multifaceted professional odyssey that cardiothoracic surgeons embark upon, beginning with the transformative period of residency and fellowship, advancing through the dynamic and diverse landscape of early- and mid-career surgeons, and culminating in the contemplative years of alternative to clinical medicine and into retirement.

Although no two surgeons are the same, this issue stands to be a comprehensive guide for common themes and landmark moments that occur throughout one's professional lifespan. This is not merely a reference; rather, it is a scholarly companion tailored for those who have chosen the challenging but rewarding path of cardiothoracic surgery. Through meticulous exploration, it seeks to illuminate the nuanced stages that characterize a career within this demanding discipline.

This unique issue is enriched by the voices and experiences of expert cardiothoracic surgeons—ranging from early to late in their careers–whose journeys serve as beacons of knowledge. Their narratives offer profound insights into the intricacies and nuances of cardiothoracic surgery, complemented by practical strategies for professional growth and resilience in the face of professional and personal challenges. Within these pages, the reader will encounter real-life stories from our esteemed contributing authors, whose experiences and insights provide invaluable guidance. Among these pages, you will discover strategies for personal and professional growth, tips for maintaining a harmonious work-life balance, and sage advice on how to adeptly navigate the ever-evolving landscape of modern cardiothoracic surgery. As you journey through these articles, remember that a career is not merely a series of milestones and achievements but a continuous process of learning and adaptation. The insights within these pages shall serve as your intellectual compass, guiding you through the dynamic seas of your professional lifespan.

"The Professional Lifespan: From Residency to Retirement" aspires to be a professional handbook—a starting point for self-reflection, a foundation for achieving longevity and fulfillment in one's career, and a repository of insightful guidance for

Thorac Surg Clin 34 (2024) xv–xvi
https://doi.org/10.1016/j.thorsurg.2023.09.003
1547-4127/24/© 2023 Published by Elsevier Inc.

the aspiring and established cardiothoracic surgeon alike.

Jinny S. Ha, MD, MHS
The Johns Hopkins School of Medicine
Division of Thoracic Surgery
Department of Surgery
600 North Wolfe Street, Blalock 240
Baltimore, MD 21287, USA

Stephen C. Yang, MD, FACS, MAMSE
The Johns Hopkins School of Medicine
Division of Thoracic Surgery
Department of Surgery
600 North Wolfe Street, Blalock 240
Baltimore, MD 21287, USA

E-mail addresses:
jha1@jhmi.edu (J.S. Ha)
syang@jhmi.edu (S.C. Yang)

Finding the Right Mentor

Fatima G. Wilder, MD, MSc[a],*, Jason J. Han, MD[b]

KEYWORDS

- Mentor • Sponsor • Cardiothoracic surgery

KEY POINTS

- Mentorship is an essential component of a successful career in cardiothoracic surgery.
- Finding a mentor and creating a successful mentor–mentee relationship requires introspection, appropriate alignment of goals, open communication, and regular feedback.
- In cardiothoracic surgery, there are many resources available to help members of the community find and maintain successful mentoring relationships.

INTRODUCTION

The concept of a mentor originated from The Odyssey, the epic Greek poem that tells the story of Odysseus' circuitous and challenging return journey home in the aftermath of the fall of Troy. At the onset of the war, Odysseus was said to have entrusted his son, Telemachus, with his friend, Mentor, who offered to provide his guidance and support. The concept of mentorship has since been integrated into modern society and, in particular, within the medical profession as part of the Hippocratic Oath, given its emphasis on teaching.[1]

MENTORSHIP IN CARDIOTHORACIC SURGERY

In pragmatic terms, a mentor is usually a senior member within the same specialty who serves as a guide for younger or less-experienced members.[2] Mentorship is an essential function of any organized profession, especially one that is as similar to an apprenticeship as cardiothoracic surgery and may pertain to professional, educational, as well as personal matters. Several studies have demonstrated the necessity of mentorship in optimizing career satisfaction and success, as well as in reducing burnout and attrition, especially during training.[3] In a series of studies in adolescent medicine and pediatrics, 95% of respondents identified the presence of a mentor as important to their training[4] and 16% believed that the presence

of mentorship was the most important aspect of their training experience.[5,6] The benefits are long term, influencing career trajectories. The influence of mentorship on retention and career longevity is especially evident in academia, where the presence of a mentor has been associated with nearly doubling faculty retention rates.[7] Physicians with mentors are more likely to receive appropriate career guidance and find themselves in a position to act on it. This results in better performance across various metrics of success, including increased academic and scientific productivity. Mentorship was also significantly associated with success in research completion and the ability to obtain funding in several studies examined.[7]

Mentorship, however, is neither a one-way street nor a passive process. Mentees bear as much of the responsibility for the success or failure of these relationships. Poorly defined goals, a lack of clear expectations, communication failures, and failure of mentees to follow-up or deliver on promised work are some of the factors that create unnecessary breakdowns in mentoring relationships.[8–10] Success relies on open communication, honest and frequent reflection, professionalism, and appropriate prioritization of tasks and responsibilities.

Mentorship Versus Sponsorship

There are several terms that may be used in reference to mentorship, but have different meanings

[a] Division of Thoracic Surgery, Department of Surgery, Brigham and Women's Hospital, 15 Francis Street, Boston, MA 02115, USA; [b] Division of Cardiovascular Surgery, Department of Surgery, University of Pennsylvania, 3400 Civic Center Boulevard East Pavilion, 2nd Floor, Philadelphia, PA 19104, USA
* Corresponding author. Division of Thoracic Surgery, 15 Francis Street, Boston, MA 02115.
E-mail address: fwilder@bwh.harvard.edu

Thorac Surg Clin 34 (2024) 1–7
https://doi.org/10.1016/j.thorsurg.2023.08.010
1547-4127/24/Published by Elsevier Inc.

Table 1
Definitions of mentorship and associated terms

	Term
Mentorship	An individual, typically more experienced in a given domain, provides advice and support to a mentee as part of an informal or formal connection based on mutual consent
Sponsorship	When an individual, typically in a position of power or authority, uses their social capital to advocate on behalf of another person. This can involve placing the reputation of the sponsor on the line
Coaching	A performance and goal-oriented process designed to achieve specific outcomes or metrics
Role-modeling	An individual serves as an exemplar of positive (or negative) behaviors for another individual to emulate or avoid

Recreated from Stephens et al.[2]

(**Table 1**). Of these, it is important to make a distinction between 2 terms that are often used interchangeably: a mentor versus a sponsor. Sponsorship is defined as advocacy by powerful senior leaders on behalf of a junior that is critical for career advancement. Sponsorship is distinct from mentorship in that it involves advocacy on the junior's behalf that puts the sponsor's reputation at risk.[2] Sponsorship involves the sponsor taking a more active role, with the sponsor serving as an advocate for promotion or nomination with a focus on leadership development. Sponsorship is more transactional and can be of particular importance later in a career.[11]

However, mentorship occurs when there is a personal commitment of the mentor to the mentee's growth. The mentor takes an expressed interest in counseling their protégé and providing information and counseling as part of the expectation of ongoing support and guidance.[6,12]

Throughout one's career, there will likely be a need for both mentors and sponsors. The same person may simultaneously fulfill the role of a mentor and a sponsor, depending on the circumstances. The distinction between these 2 terms is not meant to pose any logistical barriers or complications. The most important thing is that both parties are clear on each other's role and expectations.

Finding a Mentor

Connecting with a mentor is a multifactorial process without a single correct formula. An individual may choose to seek out one mentor or many mentors across various domains. The ideal mentor, depending on the circumstances, may be a trainee, a junior attending, a senior attending, or a retired surgeon. The mentor may or may not share an academic or research focus, or may not

have one at all. Ultimately, it is not a relationship with fixed stipulations. Rather, it is a dynamic relationship where both parties' stages of careers, needs, and ambitions continually grow; therefore, a mutual understanding of flexibility is an essential aspect.

Yet, there are certain characteristics that are more conducive to finding mentorship early on. Experience and literature on mentoring suggest that a good mentor is genuine, accomplished, accessible, attentive, motivating, and accountable.[7] Reich and colleagues described ideal mentors as being easy to work with, being within a similar subspecialty, working in a similar area of research, having a good reputation, and working in the "ideal" work environment.[3] Good mentors are active listeners that allow healthy independence for their mentees. However, they are involved enough to provide the necessary guidance and to give honest and effective feedback. Good mentors must avoid conflicts of interest with any personal goals or supervisory roles, and understand the mentee's internal motivators.

Trainees should seek out mentors early on in their careers, and first look for potential mentors within their own institutions or networks. Their availability and proximity may immediately enable a plethora of clinical, educational, and research collaborations. The mentor and mentee can, both in person or virtually, meet on a regular basis. These mentors will intuitively understand the culture and the setup of the institution and will be able to offer valuable insights on navigating its associated challenges. They will be able to help the mentee establish a realistic career roadmap, play a pivotal role in networking, and connect the mentee to productive research databases and projects without any significant logistical hurdles.

Simultaneously, it is important to also consider seeking out mentors from outside of one's

Table 2
Current mentorship opportunities in cardiothoracic surgery (CTS)

Host Organization	Programs/Scholarships of Interest
Society of Thoracic Surgeons (STS)	Looking to the Future Scholarship
American Association for Thoracic Surgery (AATS)	Member for a Day Program Honoring Our Mentors Program
Women in Thoracic Surgery (WTS)	WTS Mentorship Program Carpenter Scholarship Thistlethwaite Scholarship
Thoracic Surgery Foundation	Various research, educational, and service grants
Western Thoracic Surgical Association (WTSA)	WTSA Traveling Fellowship & Mentorship Program
Southern Thoracic Surgical Association	James W. Brooks Scholarship & Diversity Scholarship
Thoracic Surgery Directors Association (TSDA)	
Thoracic Surgery Residents Association (TSRA)	Traveling Fellowship
Thoracic Surgery Medical Students Association (TSMA)	Mentorship programs for application cycles and students from underrepresented backgrounds
Association of Black Cardiovascular and Thoracic Surgeons (ABCTS)	ABCTS Pipeline program

This table serves as a starting point, and it is not meant to be comprehensive.

institution or immediate network.[8,13,14] In the era of virtual collaborations and social media, these relationships have become relatively common, and productive. These mentors may offer deeper insights into specific areas of expertise that may not be available locally, and provide a connection to various outside networks, whether it be geographically or demographically. It is also important to acknowledge that many medical students or trainees (eg, general surgery residents) interested in applying into a highly specialized field, such as cardiothoracic surgery, may come from institutions without their own cardiothoracic surgery programs. They may, therefore, find it necessary to connect with mentors from other institutions to set up elective rotations, receive recommendation letters, or to participate in research projects. Those interested in mentorship can identify potential mentors through virtual networking sessions, webinars, publications, or even social media accounts, and respectfully reach out to them via email. One can also meet these individuals at national meetings, many of which have dedicated sessions and programs for establishing mentorship. Through outside mentors, they may obtain general advice related to the field as well as information regarding specific programs. Existing colleagues and mentors may be helpful in recommending certain individuals as potential mentors, based on their personal experiences.

Various organizations have formal mentorship programs and scholarships that help match mentees with mentors. Several are listed in **Table 2**. Although not all programs may have official scholarships or mentorship programs established, their members are often likely a good source for direct mentorship or referral to a potential mentor based on the mentee's interests and stage in their career.

THORACIC SURGERY RESIDENTS ASSOCIATION

The TSRA was established in 1997 as the trainee-led extension of the TSDA. Its mission is to represent and meet the educational interests of current and future cardiothoracic surgery residents. The organization is led by an executive committee of elected members from traditional and integrated cardiothoracic surgery programs across the United States and maintains a nonprofit status. Although its functions span across education, research, advocacy, and communication, one of its key strengths is its facilitation of networking and mentorship opportunities. Trainees can find mentorship through the TSRA in several ways.

1. Trainees can participate in a variety of projects such as podcasts (eg, interviews), webinars, and publications (eg, textbooks, online

resources, and articles) under the guidance of faculty mentors. Trainees can either respond to calls-for-participation, which are regularly distributed via the TSRA website or the newsletter, or reach out to the TSRA executive committee with novel project ideas or topics. Trainees can also apply to become a part of the executive committee, or choose to serve as a general member on one of its committees (ie, Projects Committee, Educations Committee, Membership Committee, and so forth) depending on their interests and availability. Relationships developed through these interactions may organically lead to future, recurrent professional collaborations.

2. Trainees can attend in-person and virtual networking sessions hosted by the TSRA, notably at national society meetings (eg, STS, AATS), where they can meet colleagues and mentors who share similar professional or personal interests.

3. As representatives of, or through networks developed via the TSRA, trainees can begin to serve on national committees where they can encounter leaders in the field and help provide trainees' perspectives.

In addition to seeking mentors, trainees can also begin to function as mentors to junior residents and medical students through their involvement in the TSRA, especially in their collaboration with the TSMA, described in the next session.

THORACIC SURGERY MEDICAL STUDENTS ASSOCIATION

The TSMA was founded in 2020 by a group of medical students and faculty/resident advisors to bring together and to help prepare students interested in careers in cardiothoracic surgery. The organization has been especially helpful in meeting peers and serving as mentors to students whose early exposure to the field is limited by personal and institutional proximity to mentors. Students, especially those from nontraditional backgrounds, had a difficult time obtaining information and advice on the current landscape of the field, on how to determine if the specialty is the right fit for them, the array of available training pathways—and their commonalities as well as their differences. A major topic for many of these students was surrounding how to become a competitive applicant. Similar to the TSRA, the TSMA offers various opportunities to work on projects (eg, webinars and research) that organically facilitate collaboration with residents, fellows, and attending surgeons, as well as networking events. Students can become involved

in the organization early on by reaching out to the organization, getting involved in committees, and eventually helping lead it.

OTHER CONSIDERATIONS IN MENTORSHIP
Assigned Versus Organic

Although many organizations offer opportunities to attend national and regional meetings to network with potential mentors, finding the right mentor is still an organic process. In general, studies have found that there is increased mentee satisfaction when they are able to choose their mentors, and vice versa, rather than being assigned by a program.[2,3,15] Mentees may first begin this process by having conversations with their peers and colleagues. When they voice their specific questions or needs, they may discover certain contacts who may provide the guidance they need, either by advice or by example. These mentor–mentee relationships are more likely to be durable and mutually insightful. Unlike assigned mentorship programs, there is also more likely to be a better fit accounting for various personalities, and working styles.

Formal Versus Informal

Mentoring relationships can be formal or informal and may change as the relationship grows. Informal mentorship is usually focused on specific needs that the mentee identifies.[1,16] They may not have established times to check in or clear goals but rather need the dynamic needs of the mentee primarily. Formal mentorships usually arise within an organized manner or through a formal program (training, departmental, career development award, and so forth). In formal relationships, there are typically specific goals that should be achieved and may be affiliated with a specific timeline,[17] thus enforcing a sense of accountability.[18]

Individual Versus Group

One-on-one mentoring, as the name implies, involves a single mentor and mentee.[18] Group mentoring provides the option of having multiple mentors to guide an individual mentee or several mentees at once. This allows for multiple views, areas of expertise, and flexibility in things such as scheduling. In the era of virtual interactions, group mentorships can allow individuals from multiple, distant institutions to provide support for an individual or group.

Diversity and Identity

Other more personal factors that are important to consider when establishing and maintaining a mentor–mentee relationship are age, gender, family status, culture, race, and more. Although these factors are not meant to be exclusive, there are worthwhile considerations to bear in mind regarding how they may affect the relationship. When considering gender, a study reported that during a 2-year period, more men were promoted even though more women reported having mentors. Clearly, navigating gender differences at the workplace is a highly complex process that effective mentorship should encapsulate. Awareness of this disparity can help maintain a priority of encouraging sponsorship and actively pursuing advancement opportunities for women.[19] Especially on the subject of family planning, it is important for applicants, trainees, and even faculty members to seek mentorship and support on this meaningful, yet complex process. Although the profession has, at one point in history, viewed a busy surgical career to be incompatible with an engaged family life, there has been considerable research and conversation aimed at shifting this paradigm toward greater inclusivity. Both trainees and educators alike perceive a significant need for improvement in the current system. Program directors reported that sociopolitical, cultural, and fiscal constraints pose obstacles in supporting pregnant residents.[20] In a survey of surgical residents, about a third of those who had or were expecting children during training did not feel supported in taking parental leave or in general by the faculty in their programs. Lack of policy, personnel, and flexibility in schedule were common obstacles to pursuing parental leave.[21] Moreover, in a different survey study, the majority of female surgical residents believed their work schedule adversely affected their and their fetuses' health. The majority also believed their duration of maternity leave to be inadequate.[22] Certainly, considered together, this topic does and will increasingly pose a major area of need for mentorship for all surgeons.

Across ages, it is important that the mentor be cognizant of the values and expectations of their mentee because they may vary in different generations.[23] For example, an article in the Harvard Business Review highlighted that millennials (born 1977–1997) desire jobs that will fulfill them personally; are an integral part of their lives; allow them to collaborate, make new friends, and learn new skills; and connect them to a larger social purpose.[24] These personality or perspective differences will affect the mentoring relationship and should be kept in mind when communicating or setting goals.

Racial differences are another important factor to consider in the mentoring relationship. Cardiothoracic surgery remains a white-male dominated specialty across all career stages,[25,26] although we have seen a gradual trend toward increasing diversity in recent years. In an article published in 2006, it was reported that minorities have greater difficulty gaining access to mentors. Moreover, when available mentors are generally White men, it can introduce interracial dynamics into the mentoring relationship.[24] During the years, the conversations around race-related issues have become more commonplace, and it is not unusual for institutions to now have entities specifically focused on "Diversity, Equity, and Inclusion." As a result, many resources are now available for both the mentor and mentee to call upon in navigating their relationship. Overall, it is fundamentally important to maintain open communication and create a trusting mentoring relationship where the mentor and mentee can openly discuss racial issues, sensitivities, and realities.[27,28]

SELECTING A MENTOR (AND MAKING THE MOST OUT OF MENTOR–MENTEE RELATIONSHIP)

Before asking individuals to serve as one's mentor, introspection is an important first step.[7] To make the most of these encounters, each mentee can prepare by outlining their personal and professional values and passions because they relate to their short-term and long-term goals. Mentees can prepare for meetings by gathering information on their current circumstances and options. This process will help mentees ultimately seek advice that is more specific and actionable, and in this regard, mentees can generate much of the initiative to develop the relationship.

It is important to recognize that the mentee's needs may change with time, so it is necessary to revisit one's goals at regular intervals. The needs of a mentee often depend on what stage one is in their career.[2] For example, junior residents were slightly more likely than senior residents to value mentors as role models (90% vs 82%, $P = .042$), whereas senior residents found their mentors more impactful in technical training, job counseling, and societal involvement (differences of 15%–30%). Similarly, a 2014 survey completed by 55 recent thoracic surgery residency graduates taking the American Board of Thoracic Surgery oral examination highlighted other important needs: 25% of respondents indicated that they did not receive sufficient mentoring advice to make sound career decisions and 84% believed that formal mentoring programs would have been valuable.[28,29]

The mentee should be upfront in asking the desired mentor if they will have time to foster and support the relationship. Also be honest with each potential mentor regarding the intention of meeting with several different individuals before establishing a relationship, and follow up appropriately when a final decision has been made. Once the relationship is established, it is beneficial to outline the purpose and goals of the relationship, the plan for scheduled meetings, and the responsibilities and expectations of each member of the group.[7] If there are specific things the mentee is seeking from the relationship (ie, networking, help with the job search, research involvement, and so forth), these should be stated in advance. It is also important to demonstrate a humble growth mindset by welcoming and acting on constructive feedback.

This method will likely lead to the selection of multiple mentors. They may serve in a mentorship role on a one-on-one basis, or become part of the mentees "mentorship committee" with whom they meet on a scheduled basis. Meetings should be held regularly and the mentor/mentee should avoid cancellations. Before all meetings with mentors, the mentee can consider having a written agenda that is shared ahead of time. Each agenda should include realistic short-term and long-term goals. This is essential for accountability and will ultimately enhance productivity. Even if the mentee does not think they have anything completed to share at the meeting, it provides an opportunity to check-in and course-correct if the mentee is going off track.

SUMMARY

Mentorship is a vital component of a successful career. Barring the rare serendipitously successful mentor–mentee relationship, it takes time to build and maintain a successful partnership. The skills inherent to being a good mentor and mentee are not automatic but rather must be learned and honed over time. Whatever stage one finds themselves in, it is important to have ongoing reflection. Consider pursuing the concept of "mosaic mentorship" that encourages mentees to integrate various mentorship models and strategies in order to ensure the best mentor and format is selected for the issue at hand while recognizing the evolution of their needs over time. It is more likely that throughout one's career, with the anticipated changes in goals, institutions and experience, there will be a need for multiple mentors. Whether in sequence or simultaneously, a variety of mentors will allow for the mentee to explore a conglomerate of learning strategies, call on a wide variety of experiences and skill sets, and perspectives.[18] Self-reflection and dynamic goal

setting are central to successful mentorship experiences at all stages of training, from medical school all the way through early career and even in established career stages. It requires investment but with real commitment comes the opportunity to build lasting relationships and establish a successful and rewarding career.

CLINICS CARE POINTS

- Literature on mentoring suggests that a good mentor is genuine, accomplished, accessible, attentive, motivating, and accountable.
- Poorly defined goals, a lack of clear expectations, communication failures, and failure of mentees to follow-up or deliver on promised work are some of the factors that create unnecessary breakdowns in mentoring relationships.[8–10]
- Those interested in mentorship can identify and meet potential mentors through email, virtual networking sessions, webinars, publications, or even social media accounts.
- Consider pursuing the concept of "mosaic mentorship" that encourages mentees to integrate various mentorship models and strategies in order to ensure the best mentor and format is selected for the issue at hand while recognizing the evolution of their needs over time.

DISCLOSURE

The authors have no disclosures.

REFERENCES

1. Ambrosetti A, Davis S. Mentor. M/C Journal 2016; 19(2). https://doi.org/10.5204/mcj.1103.
2. Stephens EH, Goldstone AB, Amy G, et al. Appraisal of Mentorship in Cardiothoracic Surgery Training. J ThoracCardiovas Surg 2018;156(6):2216–23.
3. Reich HJ, Lou X, Alexander A, et al. "Mentorship effectiveness in cardiothoracic surgical training. Annals Thorac Surg 2021;112(2):645–51.
4. Berk RA, Berg J, Mortimer R, et al. Measuring the effectiveness of faculty mentoring relationships. Acad Med 2005;80:66–71.
5. Lebastchi AH, Yuh DD. Nationwide survey of US integrated 6-year cardiothoracic surgical residents. J Thorac Cardiovasc Surg 2014;148:401–7.
6. Higgins R. Overcoming bias in surgery: the role of mentorship and sponsorship. Available at: https://www.youtube. com/watch?v^1/$_4$qXrVe8Y9Vvc. Accessed June 15, 2020.

7. Odell DD, Edwards M, Fuller S, et al. The art and Science of mentorship in cardiothoracic surgery: a systematic review of the literature. Annal Thorac Surg 2022;113(4):1093–100.

8. Entezami P, Franzblau LE, Chung KC. Mentorship in surgical training: a systematic review. Hand (N Y) 2012;7:30–6.

9. Sanfey H, Hollands C, Gantt NL. Strategies for building an effective mentoring relationship. Am J Surg 2013;206:714718.

10. Palepu A, Friedman RH, Barnett RC, et al. Junior faculty members' mentoring relationships and their professional development in U.S. medical schools. Acad Med 1998;73:318323.

11. Ayyala MS, Skarupski K, Bodurtha JN, et al. Mentorship is not enough: exploring sponsorship and its role in career advancement in academic medicine. Acad Med 2019;94:94–100.

12. Britt LD. Mentorship/sponsorship and leadership in academic surgery: similarities and differences. In: Scoggins C, Pollock R, Pawlik T, editors. *Surgical mentorship and leadership. Success in academic surgery.* Cham, Switzerland: Springer; 2018. p. 67–80.

13. Chopra V, Saint S. Mindful mentorship. Healthc (Amst) 2020;8:100390.

14. Zhang LM, Ellis RJ, Ma M, et al. Prevalence, types, and sources of bullying reported by US general surgery residents in 2019. JAMA 2020;323:2093–5.

15. Yamada K, Slanetz PJ, Boiselle PM. Perceived benefits of a radiology resident mentoring program: Comparison of residents with self-selected Vs assigned mentors. Can Assoc Radiol J 2014;65(2). https://doi.org/10.1016/j.carj.2013.04.001.

16. Lentz E, Allen TD. Reflections on naturally occurring mentoring relationships. In: Allen TD, Eby LT, editors. The Blackwell Handbook of mentoring: a multiple perspectives approach. Malden (MA): Blackwell; 2007. p. 159–62.

17. Kwan T, Lopez-Real F. Mentors' perceptions of their roles in mentoring student teachers. Asia Pac J Teach Educ 2005;33(3):275–87.

18. Khatchikian AD, Chahal BS, Kielar A. Mosaic Mentoring: Finding the Right Mentor for the Issue at Hand. Abdominal Radiology 2021;46(12):5480–4.

19. Ibarra H, Carter NM, Silva C. Why men still get more promotions than women. Harv Bus Rev 2010;1–6. Reprint R1009F.

20. Castillo-Angeles M, Smink DS, Rangel EL. Perspectives of US General Surgery Program Directors on Cultural and Fiscal Barriers to Maternity Leave and Postpartum Support During Surgical Training. JAMA Surgery 2021;156(7):647.

21. Altieri MS, Arghavan Salles, Bevilacqua Lisa A, et al. Perceptions of Surgery Residents About Parental Leave During Training. JAMA Surgery 2019;154(10):952.

22. Rangel EL, Smink DS. Manuel Castillo-Angeles, Gifty Kwakye, Marguerite Changala, Adil H. Haider, and Gerard M. Doherty. "Pregnancy and Motherhood During Surgical Training. JAMA Surgery 2018;153(7):644.

23. McNulty EJ. Can you manage different generations? Harvard Business School Working Knowledge for Business Leaders, Reprinted from: It's time to rethink what you think you know about managing people. Harvard Management Update February 2006;11.

24. Meister JC, Willyerd K. Mentoring millennials. Harv Bus Rev 2010;88(5):68–72.

25. Olive JK, Yost CC, Robinson JA, et al. Demographics of Current and Aspiring Integrated Six-Year Cardiothoracic Surgery Trainees. Ann Thorac Surg 2023;115(3):771–7.

26. Olive JK, Mansoor S, Simpson K, et al. Demographic Landscape of Cardiothoracic Surgeons and Residents at United States Training Programs. Ann Thorac Surg 2022;114(1):108–14.

27. Ely RJ, Meyerson DE, Davidson MN. Rethinking political correctness. Harv Bus Rev 2006;84:78–87.

28. Thomas, DA. The truth about mentoring minorities: Race matters. Harvard Business Review. 2001; 79: 98-107. https://bwhmentoringtoolkit.partners.org/mentoring-across-differences-race-culture-gender-generation/readings-and-articles/. Accessed April 21 2023.

29. Chu D, Vaporciyan AA, Iannettoni MD, et al. Are there gaps in current thoracic surgery residency training programs? Ann Thorac Surg 2016;101:2350–5.

Advanced Fellowships After Training: Super or Not?

Jennifer L. Perri, MD, MBA[a], Tom C. Nguyen, MD[b],*

KEYWORDS

• Surgical education • Structural heart • Transcatheter therapy • Minimally invasive surgery

KEY POINTS

- The main reasons to pursue super fellowship are to obtain a specialized skillset, improve candidacy for a job, and/or gain repetition in routine cases.
- The application process is individual to the program and a list of programs offered previously is published herein.
- Common tracks for super fellowship: aortic surgery, structural heart, minimally invasive coronary, minimally invasive valve, mechanical circulatory support/transplant, congenital surgery, and thoracic surgical oncology.
- A subset of trainees will need to complete additional training, that is, super fellowship, if certain skillsets are desired.

BACKGROUND

"Super fellowship" following cardiothoracic residency has garnered increased attention in the past 10 to 20 years, particularly with specialized technology and skill in the arenas of minimally invasive and robotic surgery, transcatheter interventions, and transplant.[1,2] However, a decision to pursue additional training after 6 to 8 years of clinical operative experience incurs an opportunity cost in both time and money. In a recent survey study of 261 graduates,[2] 40% of trainees pursued additional years of training. Participants on online medical forums such as Student Doctor Network commonly cite reasons for pursuing additional training as (1) acquisition of a specialized skillset, (2) improved candidacy for a job, and (3) additional practice for improved proficiency.[3] There is a new research attempting to objectively determine why applicants pursue additional training. In 2022 and 2023, annual meetings of the Society of Thoracic Surgery (STS) and American Association of Thoracic Surgery (AATS) featured invited lectures on the topic of additional specialized training.[4,5] Herein, we provide an overview of the existing data related to cardiac, congenital, and thoracic "super fellowship." The objective data are limited, therefore in certain circumstances the information is taken from blogs, web sites, and personal anecdotes to provide the most comprehensive review.

EMERGING TECHNOLOGIES

Cardiothoracic surgery since its inception has been advanced by technology and innovation. Double lumen endotracheal tubes pioneered in the 1930s to 1950s paved the way for single lung ventilation,[6] which allowed for the advent of minimally invasive lung resection techniques. Cardiopulmonary bypass first safely implemented in man in 1953[7] allowed for coronary bypass in the late 1950s and valve replacement in the 1960s. Innovation, now more than ever is crucial to offering similar interventions through smaller incisions or offering lifesaving surgery to patients previously deemed inoperable. There exist 2 types of innovation—sustaining and disruptive. Although sustaining innovation works to improve existing devices and framework, disruptive innovation is new and different.[8] Minimally invasive interventions in

[a] Division of Cardiovascular and Thoracic Surgery, Duke University Medical Center, Durham, NC, USA;
[b] Division of Adult Cardiothoracic Surgery, UCSF Medical Center, 500 Parnassus Avenue, MUW 405, Box 0118, San Francisco, CA 94143, USA
* Corresponding author. 500 Parnassus Avenue, MUW 405, Box 0118, San Francisco, CA 94143.
E-mail address: tom.c.nguyen@gmail.com

Thorac Surg Clin 34 (2024) 9–15
https://doi.org/10.1016/j.thorsurg.2023.08.001

cardiothoracic surgery have typically been adopted as disruptive technology, completely unlike previous techniques and requiring additional skills to master. In that realm, it is challenging to incorporate minimally invasive surgery and new devices in routine training. In cardiac surgery transcatheter aortic valve replacement (TAVR), transcatheter edge-to-edge repair (TEER), branched thoracic endovascular aortic repair (TEVAR), minimally invasive coronary artery bypass grafting (MICS CABG), Impella (Abiomed, Danvers, MA), and continuous centrifugal flow left ventricular assist device, that is, HeartMate III (Abbott Laboratories, Lake Forest, IL), did not exist in the prior century. In thoracic surgery, the first video-assisted thoracoscopic surgery (VATS) lobectomy took place in 1991[9] and the first robotic-assisted thoracoscopic surgery (RATS) lobectomy in 2002.[10] As the field becomes more complex, with specialized techniques and new technology having a role in day-to-day surgery, there is clearly a need for some percentage of trainees to obtain specialized training. In a recent publication on future direction in training, the authors both minimally invasive cardiac surgeons opine "Whether transcatheter therapies or MICS, the biggest challenge arguably remains the additional learning curves that must be mastered … expertise is required in traditional surgical skills, imaging, and catheter-based skills to fully implement these new techniques."[11] Likely these techniques cannot be mastered with standard training alone. In these circumstances super fellowship seems crucial.

CURRENT TRAINING PARADIGMS

The American Board of Thoracic Surgery (ABTS) established in 1948 has offered a traditional modality of training since its inception, that is, 5 years of general surgery followed by 2 to 3 years of cardiothoracic training. Currently, the ABTS offers 4 "pathways to certification": (1) traditional track, (2) 4/3 fast track, (3) integrated cardiothoracic residency, (4) integrated vascular surgery residency followed by traditional cardiothoracic residency.[12] Residents must achieve proficiency in both thoracic and cardiovascular procedures, and as both primary and assistant surgeon. Simulation has been shown to reduce operative time in coronary anastomoses, and there is a mandatory 20 hour simulation training in the ABTS case requirements.[13] To remain up to date with rapidly changing technique and technology, some surgeons have advocated for "disease-specific fellowships", that is, super fellowship. This concept has not yet been adopted by the ABTS but has been suggested at national meetings and in journal publications.[4,5,11]

LOGISTICS—HOW TO FIND A SUPER FELLOWSHIP

Unlike residency training sponsored by the Accreditation Council for the Graduate Medical Education (ACGME), super fellowships are not posted to the Electronic Residency Application Service web site. Thus, determining current offerings training openings is a more esoteric process. A list of institutions that have historically offered structured additional training is listed in **Table 1**. These institutions have posted on CTSNet, Thoracic Surgery Directors Association, or their hospital web sites. An additional year of non-ACGME training is still subject to the rules and regulations of the Graduate Medical Education (GME) board at the affiliated hospital. For example, "super fellows" remain under hours regulations of the hospital GME. The applications typically require 3 letters of recommendation and USMLE scores; deadlines can be variable but most common is a September deadline in advance of an August start date the following year.

WHY ADDED TRAINING?

In the most comprehensive survey study to date published in 2021, surgeons from the University of Michigan emailed a 10 question survey to all CT surgery graduates between 2008 and 2019, 776 graduates total.[2] A total of 261 responses were obtained, with a response rate of 34%. The main findings are distilled to 2 areas, type of training and the reason listed as the primary motivation for additional training. In terms of type, 35% pursued congenital, 22% mechanical circulatory support (MCS)/transplant, 16% aortic, 3% valve with 12% of survey respondents writing in a field that was thoracic in nature. When asked reasons, the most common was congenital (35%), inadequate training (28%), and requirement for a job (24%). Regarding pathway, the findings showed those who completed general surgery and a traditional 2 to 3 year residency were more likely to complete additional training than those who completed an integrated residency. The authors did not conduct an analysis by gender. This study may have an underlying response bias because those who pursued extra training may have been more likely to answer the survey out of personal interest. When respondents who pursued additional training for congenital fellowship were excluded, 26% of trainees who entered adult cardiac or adult thoracic surgery pursued a super fellowship. Those caveats aside, this study establishes that trainees seek extra training typically because of a desire to obtain a higher level skillset and/or because of perceived deficiencies in training.

Table 1
Available super fellow positions as posted on CTSNet, Thoracic Surgery Directors Association, and individual hospital web sites

List of Current Super Fellowships in Cardiac, Thoracic, and Congenital Surgery	
Aortic Surgery	*Mechanical Circulatory Support/Transplant*
Memorial Hermann Texas Medical Center	Baylor University Medical Center/BSW Health (Dallas, TX)
Baylor/Texas Heart Institute	Brigham and Women's Hospital
Cleveland Clinic	Cedar-Sinai Medical System
Duke University Hospital	Cleveland Clinic
Emory University Hospital	Mayo Clinic
Mount Sinai Hospital	New York Presbyterian/Columbia
Northwestern Memorial Hospital	Northwestern Memorial Hospital
New York Presbyterian/Weill Cornell	Stanford Medical Center
Toronto General Hospital	Temple University Hospital
University of Alabama	University of California Los Angeles (Ronald Reagan UCLA Medical Center)
University of Michigan	University of Chicago
University of Pennsylvania	University of Michigan
	University of Pittsburgh Medical Center
Structural Heart	University of Utah Hospital
Brigham and Women's Hospital	
Emory University Hospital	*Thoracic Minimally Invasive*
New York/Columbia Presbyterian	Duke University Hospital
New York University	Mayo Clinic
	MD Anderson Cancer Center
Minimally Invasive Coronary Artery Bypass	Memorial Sloan Kettering Cancer Center
Lankenau Medical Center	Temple Fox Chase Cancer Center
Mount Sinai Medical Center	University of Pittsburgh Medical Center
University of Chicago	
	Congenital—see ACGME-accredited programs
Minimally Invasive Valve Repair	
Baylor College of Medicine (Houston, TX)	
Cleveland Clinic	
Emory University Hospital	
Lenox Hill Hospital/Northwell Health	
New York University Langone Health	

REVIEW OF SUPER FELLOWSHIPS BY SUBSPECIALTY
Aortic Surgery

In the STS database the median number of type A dissections performed at an institution is 3.[14] The author's 2019 publication based on data from the Memorial Herman Health System shows a clear association between higher volume of dissections performed per surgeon and lower 30 day mortality.[15] In a 2019 article by Chen and colleagues, even when performed during a type A dissection mortality of a valve sparing root replacement was only 3.4% when performed at a center with a high volume tertiary care aortic center.[16] That is to say these experts have established that dissections have lower mortality performed at a high volume center and challenging operations such as a total arch or valve sparing root replacement have improved outcomes at these centers. The operations learned in aortic fellowship are (1) redo AVR/root replacement, (2) Zone 2 or total arch replacement, (3) valve sparing root replacement and valve repair techniques, and (4) TEVAR $\pm$ branched technique.

The topic of endovascular aortic repair is increasingly important. The first TEVAR was performed in 1992 at the Stanford Medical Center by Dr Craig Miller and Dr Michael Dake.[17] The first branched device (Gore TBE) received FDA approval in 2022.[18] Now in 2023, 2 additional thoracic branch devices are in trial in the United States (Relay Branched device, Terumo, Sunrise, FL; Endospan NEXUS, Herzlia, Israel). Survey studies have suggested trainees feel ill prepared in endovascular techniques. In a 2016, in Service Exam Survey, 52% of respondents were "uncomfortable" performing TAVR and 49% were "uncomfortable" performing TEVAR. Fifty-eight percent of respondents noted competition for cases as a main reason for lack of training.[19] Aortic super fellowship offers trainees the experience to master new devices in the endovascular domain and to perform cases such a total arch replacement or aortic valve repair that have improved results when performed by an experienced surgeon.

STRUCTURAL HEART

Approval for TAVR in prohibitive risk patients for severe aortic stenosis came from the FDA in 2011.[20] In 2017, the ACGME introduced TAVR as a graduating case requirement, with 5 cases in the primary surgeon role and 10 as assistant. In 2022 that number was increased to 20 in each role for cardiac track candidates.[21] In the aforementioned in service training survey, 78% of respondents noted difficulty with TAVR deployment.[19] Forty-five residents completed a web-based survey in a Canadian study specifically directed at trainee experience with catheter-based therapy. After a TAVR-specific rotation, only 58% reported being able to independently perform a TAVR, 35% said competition with trainees from other specialties limited their learning, and 88% said additional training should be devoted to catheter-based skills.[22] The authors have published on this subject, and feel a designated structural heart disease training pathway should be incorporated into the existing training curriculum with an increase in primary operator cases to 25.[23] Skills learned either with a more formal rotation or additional training are 3-dimensional modeling and measurements for TAVR sizing, valve in valve TAVR, transseptal access, transcaval access, percutaneous transaxillary access, BASILICA procedure, and transcatheter mitral repair/replacement. Structural heart super fellowship offers trainees not yet independent in TAVR and TEER additional operative experience and case practice in more complex anatomic situations.

MINIMALLY INVASIVE CORONARY

Off pump CABG, MICS CABG, and robotic CABG all have a substantial learning curve. Although the ROOBY trial and others have not shown a long-term mortality benefit in off pump CABG, in a large study of 186,458 patients enrolled in the STS database, when only surgeons were included who performed at least 150 off pump coronary bypass operations per 3 year period, there was a significant reduction in mortality in the off pump group.[24] In a discussion at the 2023 International Coronary Congress, Drs John Taggart, John Puskas, and Mark Ruel opined that to master off pump, all arterial, and minimally invasive methods the field requires subspecialization and designated coronary training. With respect to the learning curve in mastering these techniques, a study using the STS database noted that for robot-assisted CABG, complications were reduced after the 10th case.[25] However, in another study incorporating mid- and long-term outcomes, proficiency in this operation was achieved only after 250 to 500 cases.[26] Additional training in coronary surgery is relatively recent, to the authors' knowledge the first structured coronary artery fellowship was offered under Dr John Puskas in 2013. Minimally invasive coronary super fellowship offers the trainee high volume coronary experience in a field shown to have a steep learning curve, and where CABG outcomes are recorded in the STS Registry and in certain states publicly reported at the surgeon level.

MINIMALLY INVASIVE VALVE

Along the same vein, minimally invasive or robotic valve repair presents a similar challenge in training with a learning curve. The oft quoted Leipzig paper cites 75 to 125 cases necessary to achieve proficiency in minimally invasive mitral surgery.[27] Although minimally invasive mitral valve repair allows for less blood loss, faster recovery, and reduced post-operative pain,[28] only 23% of mitral valve surgeries are performed via a thoracotomy in the United States.[29] Several programs offer training in minimally invasive or robotic mitral valve repair. As published by the Cleveland Clinic, numerous factors go into selecting patients for a robotic approach that limits the number of patients who qualify for this operation.[30] The New York University has published excellent outcomes in robotic mitral repair with one surgeon as bedside assistant and one surgeon at the console.[31] With limited case numbers and a high degree of attending involvement, often 2 attendings, these cases require extra training to gain experience. Minimally invasive valve super fellowship offers the trainee repetition in a domain with a volume-related learning curve.

MECHANICAL CIRCULATORY SUPPORT/TRANSPLANT

In the past decade heart, transplant has increased in the United States by 71% (from 2407 in 2012–4111 in 2022), and lung transplant by 51% (from 1783 to 2692).[32–34] In a review of CTSNet career postings in the 2022 to 2023 academic year, the most commonly listed subspecialty for an academic assistant professor position was in the field of MCS/transplant.[35] In a 2017 survey study, the authors surveyed all program directors in the country overseeing a cardiothoracic surgery residency. Among respondents, 26 offered a transplant fellowship. However, of the programs with transplant super fellowship, only 56% of fellows were eligible for American Board of Surgery Examinations and only 38% went on to find a job performing heart or lung transplant. Program directors cited unpredictable work schedule and long hours as the primary reasons a career in transplant may be viewed as unfavorable.[1] With increased transplant volume since the study was published, there is likely now higher job demand in this subspecialty. In the United Kingdom, a looming shortage of transplant surgeons was identified by the government and thus a handful of surgeons were recruited for a specialized 3-month transplant fellowship. In a survey study of these participants, 7 of 8 recommended the additional training fellowship. Median satisfaction reported was 6 on a 10 point scale.[36] Transplant super fellowship offers repetition and instruction in the fastest growing subspecialty within cardiothoracic surgery, and likely is beneficial in a job search for those pursuing a career at an academic medical center.

CONGENITAL SURGERY

The first ACGME accredited fellowship in congenital surgery was approved in 2006. Then in 2009 the ABTS instituted a written and oral examination for accreditation in this subspecialty. Starting in 2023, the fellowship was transitioned to a 2 year requirement. At present, 12 programs offer an ACGME-approved fellowship. The STS began to publicly report outcomes in pediatric and congenital cardiac surgery in 2015, drawing further attention to outcomes in an already highly scrutinized field. In a 2017 survey study, respondents comment on the strengths and weaknesses of the formal congenital fellowship.[37] Thirty-five surgeons responded. Around 91% surgeons did not feel ready to operate independently at the conclusion of their training. Most commonly 3 years was

listed as the average timeframe to operate independently after graduating. Senior mentorship was listed as important by 97% of survey respondents and the most common reason for changing jobs was lack of mentorship. Despite multiple revisions to the curriculum and training paradigm, becoming independent in congenital cardiac surgery remains a challenge. This study highlights that senior mentorship at a first job is crucial.

THORACIC MINIMALLY INVASIVE FELLOWSHIP

Minimally invasive thoracic surgery took off in the 1990s with VATS lobectomy, and in 2002 the first series of robotic lobectomy was published.[10] In prior publications, it has been suggested that trainees entering with a general surgery background likely have the requisite skill set for thoracoscopic and robotic interventions.[2] However, since the approval of the first integrated program in 2001 it is not clear how that affects the training paradigm. Dr Robert Cerfolio has been a pioneer in standardizing robotic lobectomy teaching and training.[38] Even as related to robotic-assisted esophagectomy, Van der Sluis and colleagues showed with regimented instruction the learning curve can be brought down to 24 cases.[39] The AATS currently offers a robotic thoracic bootcamp to all interested trainees. Multiple avenues exist including industry sponsored courses, AATS bootcamp, and STS hands on workshops for trainees to improve their robotic skills. However, there may be variability in experience or need for high-volume practice, and in that case super fellowship will be beneficial. The cases that should be mastered in a Thoracic Minimally Invasive Fellowship include VATS lobectomy, RATS lobectomy, advanced endoscopic foregut surgery, and minimally invasive esophagectomy. These programs have historically been attractive options for surgeons coming from around the world who may not have the exposure to minimally invasive methods now pervasive in thoracic oncology in the United States. The Thoracic Minimally Invasive super fellowship offers the trainee the opportunity to master minimally invasive techniques in treatment of lung and esophageal cancer.

LOOKING TO THE FUTURE

Cardiothoracic surgery has become increasingly specialized with the advent of minimally invasive techniques, transcatheter options, and rapid growth in heart and lung transplant. Although coronary artery bypass, valve replacement, and open lung resection was the bread and butter practice of a CT surgeon as late as the 1990s, the field has become more complex. Presently a majority of assistant professor academic job postings require an area of subspecialization. The decision to pursue a super fellowship is individual and depends heavily on the skillset seeking to be mastered. Surgeons at Stanford Department of Cardiothoracic Surgery attempted to answer the question as to whether obtaining additional training led to more publications, that is, a higher H-index, or faster track to achieving full professorship. Although they found no difference comparing 78 cardiothoracic surgeons who did advanced fellowships versus 149 who did not, the study chronicled surgeons who began their attending career 1998 to 2012.[40] In recent times with rapid evolution of technology, one might imagine the results would have been drastically different. To have the skillset requisite for several of the posted open jobs, and to advance the field, it seems necessary to be "super" and in that sense complete a super fellowship.

Looking to the future, trainee case log requirements will likely have continued updates to reflect new technology, as was done for TAVR and TEVAR. Another option to adapt training to evolving techniques is to further divide training by track, as has been done for thoracic versus cardiovascular. One could imagine a third track, heart/lung transplant, being incorporated into a program. The paradigm established by the "super fellowship" seems to be advantageous, with 1 to 2 years of extra training for residents pursuing advanced level techniques. Although not ACGME accredited, the common subspecialties of super fellowship are well known by the governing boards. Perhaps if a certificate in a subspecialty was offered, it might be an additional enticement. Regardless, in a rapidly changing and complex field, obtaining a super fellowship can only serve to augment the credentials of a young surgeon starting out, seeking a first job.

DISCLOSURE

The viewpoints described in this text reflect the personal opinions of the authors and are not endorsed by the American Board of Thoracic Surgery or Thoracic Surgery Directors Association. The authors have no relevant commercial or financial conflicts of interest.

REFERENCES

1. Makdisi G, Makdisi T, Caldeira CC, et al. Surgical thoracic transplant training: Super Fellowship—Is it super? J Surg Educ 2018;75(4):1034–8.
2. Bergquist CS, Brescia AA, Watt TMF, et al. Super fellowships among cardiothoracic trainees: Prevalence and motivations. Ann Thorac Surg 2021;111(5):1724–9.
3. Non-ACGME cardiac surgery fellowships/superfellowships. Student Doctor Network Web site. Available at: https://forums.studentdoctor.net/threads/non-acgme-cardiac-surgery-fellowships-superfellowships.1322577/. Accessed June 12, 2023.
4. Chan J., Why and how to choose a super fellowship [Internet]. Presented at: 102nd AATS Annual Meeting. 2022 May 14; Boston, MA. Available at: https://www.aats.org/resources/1035. Accessed June 12, 2023.
5. Fullerton D.A., Resident education in 2028: Evolution or specialization [Unpublished lecture notes]. Presented at: STS 59th Annual Meeting. 2023 January 24; San Diego, CA.
6. Ng A, Swanevelder J. Hypoxaemia during one-lung anaesthesia. Cont Educ Anaesth Crit Care Pain 2010;10(4):117–22.
7. Stoney WS. Evolution of cardiopulmonary bypass. Circulation 2009;119(21):2844–53.
8. Christensen CM. The innovator's dilemma : when new technologies cause great firms to fail. Boston (MA): Harvard Business Review Press; 2000.
9. Roviaro G, Rebuffat C, Varoli F, et al. Video-endoscopic pulmonary lobectomy for cancer. Surg Laparosc Endosc 1992;2(3):244–7. Available at: https://www.ncbi.nlm.nih.gov/pubmed/1341539.
10. Menconi G,MA, Melfi F, Givigliano F, et al. Robotic pulmonary lobectomy early operative experience and preliminary clinical results. Eur Surg 2002;34(3):173–6. Available at: https://onlinelibrary.wiley.com/doi/abs/10.1046/j.1563-2563.2002.02042.x.
11. Abri QA, von Ballmoos MCW. Cardiovascular surgery procedural training and evaluation: Current status and future directions. Methodist DeBakey cardiovascular journal 2022;18(3):30–8. Available at: https://search.proquest.com/docview/2680242310.
12. Pathways to certification. American Board of Thoracic Surgery Web site. Available at: https://www.abts.org/ABTS/CertificationWebPages/Pathways%20to%20Certification.aspx. Updated 2023. Accessed June 25, 2023.
13. Fann JI, Calhoon JH, et al. Simulation in coronary artery anastomosis early in cardiothoracic surgical residency training: The boot camp experience. J Thorac Cardiovasc Surg 2010;139(5):1275–81. Available at: https://www.clinicalkey.es/playcontent/1-s2.0-S0022522309011453.
14. Lee TC, Kon Z, Cheema FH, et al. Contemporary management and outcomes of acute type A aortic dissection: An analysis of the STS adult cardiac surgery database. J Card Surg 2018;33(1):7–18. Available at: https://onlinelibrary.wiley.com/doi/abs/10.1111/jocs.13511.
15. Umana-Pizano JB, Nissen AP, Sandhu HK, et al. Acute type A dissection repair by high-volume vs low-volume surgeons at a high-volume aortic center. Ann Thorac Surg 2019;108(5):1330–6.

16. Rosenblum JM, Leshnower BG, Moon RC, et al. Durability and safety of david V valve-sparing root replacement in acute type A aortic dissection. J Thorac Cardiovasc Surg 2019;157(1):14–23.e1.

17. Dake MD, Miller DC, Semba CP, et al. Transluminal placement of endovascular stent-grafts for the treatment of descending thoracic aortic aneurysms. N Engl J Med 1994;331(26):1729–34. Available at: http://content.nejm.org/cgi/content/abstract/331/26/1729.

18. Federal Drug Administration. GORE TAG thoracic branch endoprosthesis. Available at: https://www.fda.gov/medical-devices/recently-approved-devices/gore-tag-thoracic-branch-endoprosthesis-p210032. Updated 2022. Accessed June 12, 2023.

19. Vardas PN, Stefanescu Schmidt AC, Lou X, et al. Current status of endovascular training for cardiothoracic surgery residents in the united states. Ann Thorac Surg 2017;104(5):1748–54.

20. Barbash IM, Waksman R. Overview of the 2011 food and drug administration circulatory system devices panel of the medical devices advisory committee meeting on the edwards SAPIEN™ transcatheter heart valve. Circulation 2012;125(3):550–5. Available at: https://www.ncbi.nlm.nih.gov/pubmed/22271848.

21. Case requirements for thoracic surgery pathways review committee for thoracic surgery . ACGME Web site. Available at: https://prod.acgme.org/globalassets/pfassets/programresources/case_requirements_for_thoracic_surgery_pathways.pdf. Updated 2022. Accessed June 12, 2023.

22. Juanda N, Chan V, Chan R, et al. Catheter-based educational experiences: A canadian survey of current residents and recent graduates in cardiac surgery. Can J Cardiol 2016;32(3):391–4.

23. Nguyen TC, Tang GHL, Nguyen S, et al. The train has left: Can surgeons still get a ticket to treat structural heart disease? J Thorac Cardiovasc Surg 2019;157(6):2369 76.e2.

24. Puskas J.D., OPCAB: Is It a Better Strategy? Presented at: STS/AATS Tech-Con 2009 and STS 45th Annual Meeting. 2009 January 24-25; San Francisco, CA.

25. Patrick WL, Iyengar A, Han JJ, et al. The learning curve of robotic coronary arterial bypass surgery: A report from the STS database. J Card Surg 2021;36(11):4178–86. Available at: https://onlinelibrary.wiley.com/doi/abs/10.1111/jocs.15945.

26. Jonsson A, Binongo J, Patel P, et al. Mastering the learning curve for robotic-assisted coronary artery bypass surgery. Ann Thorac Surg 2023;115(5):1118–25.

27. Holzhey D, Seeburger J, Misfeld M, et al. Learning minimally invasive mitral valve surgery: A cumulative sum sequential probability analysis of 3895 operations from a single high-volume center. Circulation 2013;128(5):483–91. Available at: https://www.ncbi.nlm.nih.gov/pubmed/23804253.

28. Vervoort D, Nguyen DH, Nguyen TC. When culture dictates practice: Adoption of minimally invasive mitral valve surgery. Innovations 2020;15(5):406–9. Available at: https://journals.sagepub.com/doi/full/10.1177/1556984520948644.

29. Gammie JS, Chikwe J, Badhwar V, et al. Isolated mitral valve surgery: The society of thoracic surgeons adult cardiac surgery database analysis. Ann Thorac Surg 2018;106(3):716–27.

30. Chemtob RA, Wierup P, Mick SL, et al. A conservative screening algorithm to determine candidacy for robotic mitral valve surgery. J Thorac Cardiovasc Surg 2022;164(4):1080–7.

31. Loulmet DF, Ranganath NK, Neuburger PJ, et al. Can complex mitral valve repair be performed with robotics? an institution's experience utilizing a dedicated team approach in 500 patients. Eur J Cardio Thorac Surg 2019;56(3):470–8. Available at: https://www.ncbi.nlm.nih.gov/pubmed/30753381. doi: 10.1093/ejcts/ezz029.

32. Colvin-Adams M, Smithy JM, Heubner BM, et al. OPTN/SRTR 2012 annual data report: Heart. Am J Transplant 2014;14(S1):113–38. Available at: https://onlinelibrary.wiley.com/doi/abs/10.1111/ajt.12583.

33. Valapour M, Skeans MA, Heubner BM, et al. OPTN/SRTR 2012 annual data report: Lung. Am J Transplant 2014;14(S1):139–65. Available at: https://onlinelibrary.wiley.com/doi/abs/10.1111/ajt.12584.

34. 2022 organ transplants again set annual records. UNOS Web site. Available at: https://unos.org/news/2022-organ-transplants-again-set-annual-records/. Accessed June 12, 2023.

35. Careers. CTSNet Web site. Available at: https://jobs.ctsnet.org/jobs/. Updated 2023. Accessed June 12, 2023.

36. Khoshbin E, Clark S. The national surgical training scheme in cardiothoracic transplantation: Training competent transplant surgeons in the united kingdom. Ann Surg Edu 2021;2(1):1015.

37. Mery CM, Kane LC. The ACGME fellowship in congenital cardiac surgery: The graduates' perspective. Semin Thorac Cardiovasc Surg Pediatr Card Surg Annu 2017;20:70–6. Available at: https://www.clinicalkey.es/playcontent/1-s2.0-S1092912616300072.

38. Cerfolio RJ, Cichos KH, Wei B, et al. Robotic lobectomy can be taught while maintaining quality patient outcomes. J Thorac Cardiovasc Surg 2016;152(4):991–7. Available at: https://www.clinicalkey.es/playcontent/1-s2.0-S0022522316303002.

39. van der Sluis PC, Ruurda JP, van der Horst S, et al. Learning curve for robot-assisted minimally invasive thoracoscopic esophagectomy: Results from 312 cases. Ann Thorac Surg 2018;106(1):264–71.

40. Wang H, Bajaj SS, Williams KM, et al. Impact of advanced clinical fellowship training on future research productivity and career advancement in adult cardiac surgery. Surgery 2021;169(5):1221–7.

What Is the "Right" First Job?

Rachel Kim, MD[a], Nahush A. Mokadam, MD[b],*

KEYWORDS

- Cardiothoracic surgery • Fellowship • Residency • Job application • Contract

KEY POINTS

- There are few resources available regarding the process of finding the first cardiothoracic surgeon job after training.
- Early goal-directed and mentorship-assisted preparation is integral for preparing for the job search.
- There is no single best resource available to search and apply for jobs but the cardiothoracic community and mentors are often a good place to start.
- Understanding practice type, scope, model, expectations, and team members is a good foundation during the interview period.
- Understanding the basic components of a contract will make the job search process less intimidating.

INTRODUCTION

It is a daunting task to find the "right" first job. However, the foundation of the search is similar to that of the interview and match process for residency and fellowship. Does the job opportunity have the makeup of clinical and research opportunities, case mix, support and culture that will set the trainee up to fulfill his or her early career goals? Does the position seem like a good fit? The variation occurs with (1) the mystery behind it—there are scarce resources available on the topic, and (2) the logistics: where and when to look; the interview process; the job offer and the contract. It is quite common for the first job to not be the last. That being said, this study will serve as a guide to maximize this first work experience.

DISCUSSION
Preparation

The journey to becoming a cardiothoracic surgeon requires time and dedication. The first element of finding the right first job is the preparation that has been put in throughout training. A good starting point is identifying and creating a list of personal and professional career goals. If there is a specific niche of interest, the resident should work to publish or create in that space. Along these lines, it is beneficial for the resident to attend and present at annual meetings and events that will support these goals. With this preparation, the resident's curriculum vitae (CV) should be updated on a rolling basis and reviewed with mentors. Similar to a CV, creating a "portfolio of value"[1] can be helpful. A portfolio of value displays candidate's strengths in clinical, scholarly, educational, and administrative areas (**Table 1**).

In addition to keeping an updated CV, it is helpful to write a generic cover letter that can then be modified for specific jobs the resident is interested in. This cover letter should convey information that will grab the attention of employers and that highlights important parts of the CV, skillset, or career thus far. It should also include references that the potential employer can reach out to.

a Cardiothoracic Surgery, The Ohio State University Wexner Medical Center, N-825 Doan Hall 410 West 10th Avenue, Columbus, OH 43210, USA; b Division of Cardiac Surgery, Surgical Services, Heart and Vascular Center, The Ohio State University Wexner Medical Center, N-825 Doan Hall 410 West 10th Avenue, Columbus, OH 43210, USA
* Corresponding author.
E-mail address: Nahush.Mokadam@osumc.edu

Thorac Surg Clin 34 (2024) 17–23
https://doi.org/10.1016/j.thorsurg.2023.08.009
1547-4127/24/© 2023 Elsevier Inc. All rights reserved.

Table 1
Portfolio of value

"PORTFOLIO OF VALUE"
For Medical Students, Residents, Early Career Professionals

1. Clinical Activity	• Work RVUs • Total cases • New procedures performed/learned • Specialized training (eg, robotic certification) • Accomplishments (eg, 500th transplant) • Leadership roles (eg, Director of Min Inv Surgery)
2. Scholarly Activity	• Manuscripts (accepted or published) • Editorials/Letters • Chapters • H-Index • Grants (Role, effort, $) • Clinical Trials ((Role, effort, $)) • IRBs Study Section/Grant review • Editorial responsibilities
3. Educational Activity	• National/International Talks • Regional Talks • Local Talks • Courses (Med Student courses with course #) • New Curricula (eg, simulation program) • Educational leadership roles (eg, Associate Program Director) • Mentorship of Students/Residents
4. Administrative	• Organizations • Local committees • National committees • Leadership appointments • Honors and awards • Significant process improvements (eg, implemented ERAS)

From Mokadam NA. Pro Tips for Every CT Surgeon Searching for that First Job - Part I Preparation. STS Career Resources. https://www.sts.org/resources/career-resources/blog/pro-tips-every-ct-surgeon-searching-first-job-part-i. with permission.

The various cardiothoracic organizations have online resources or sessions at annual meetings that will help jumpstart the process to finding the right first job. The Society of Thoracic Surgeons (STS) Workforce on Career Development has a web site with various resources[2] including blog posts[1,3,4] and video links to previous career advice events. Annual cardiothoracic meetings have career focused sessions (**Table 2**).[5] The American Association for Thoracic Surgery annual meeting has a Cardiothoracic Careers College. The STS has a residents' luncheon as well as a career fair. Similarly, the Western Thoracic Surgical Association has a resident symposium that provides early career and job search information.

Foundation: What Are You Looking For?

The first cardiothoracic surgery job may be many trainees' first job outside of residency and fellowship. A vital component to finding the right first job is to think critically about what one is looking for. These ideal job qualities are broken down into (1) type and scope of practice, (2) practice structure, (3) location, (4) goals and growth, and (5) support and culture.

Type of practice are categorized as academic, semiacademic, or nonacademic.[6] For academic positions, there are often clinical, research, and education components. Within academics, there are variations in the type of track available. For tenured positions, there is emphasis on academic achievement and criteria that need to be met within a certain timeframe for promotion. Tenured positions may have a separate research or education focus. For nontenured or clinical positions, there is more emphasis on clinical productivity. In semiacademic practices, there is an affiliation with an academic center, residency program, or medical school. There may be some level of engagement or teaching with trainees but often not as consistently as in an academic position. In nonacademic positions, there are generally no research responsibilities, and often times, limited medical student or resident involvement. Nonuniversity academic centers are becoming more

Table 2
Summary of conference-associated career planning resources

AATS	Annual conference, April/May	AATS/TSRA Preparing Yourself for an Academic Career	Informal session designed for Residents, Fellows, and Medical Students invested in becoming CT surgeons.
		Cardiothoracic Careers College	Day-long forum facilitated by AATS members covering salient topics pertaining to career planning.[a]
STS	Annual conference, January	Residents Symposium	Half-day forum facilitated by STS members covering early career information such as job search and transition to practice.[a]
		Residents Luncheon	Informal session designed for residents to have small-group networking opportunities with STS members.
		STS/CTSNet Career Fair	Direct opportunity for candidates and employers to connect and network.
WTSA	Annual conference, June	Residents Symposium	Half-day forum covering early career information such as job search and contract negotiation.

Abbreviations: AATS, American association for thoracic surgery; TSRA, thoracic surgery residents association; CT, cardiothoracic; STS, society of thoracic surgeons; WTSA, western thoracic surgical association.
[a] Presented material available online.
From Sterbling HM, Molena D, Rao SR, Stein SL, Litle VR. Initial report on young cardiothoracic surgeons' first job: From searching to securing and the gaps in between. The Journal of Thoracic and Cardiovascular Surgery. 2019;158(2):632-641.e3. doi:10.1016/j.jtcvs.2018.12.104; with permission.

commonplace, and do meaningfully contribute to science, education, clinical trials, and innovation.

Deciding on the scope of future practice is important as well. There are cardiac, thoracic, mixed cardiothoracic, and mixed cardiovascular positions. If an applicant wants to focus primarily on cardiac or thoracic, especially if his or her training has been primarily in one track, he or she should be cautious of opportunities that ask or require doing both or cross-covering. It is best to look for jobs that align with one's desired scope of practice. Though it is advisable to be a good partner and be available, covering more than anticipated in terms of scope of practice can lead to emergency cases or scenarios that one may be ill prepared for early on.

Beyond general scope of practice, if a candidate has specific subspecialty interests, it is important to evaluate whether a potential job has opportunities for growth or involvement in that area. However, he or she should be cautious when considering positions that want a candidate to lead or start an entirely new program (eg, starting a lung transplant or robotics program) for the first job out of training. It takes a lot of infrastructure and support to build a new program. Early on, the focus should be on starting off strong, learning the system, developing independence, and being a safe competent surgeon with good outcomes.

Practice model is another consideration. Categories include physician groups, hospital or government employed positions, and private practice groups. Single or multispecialty physician groups are typically a hybrid between hospital employed and private practice groups. These physician groups may have agreements with academic centers or health care systems. Hospital employed positions or government employed positions are the model that trainees are most familiar with. In these positions, the surgeon is a hospital employee mostly uninvolved in the business aspect of the practice. There is often more financial stability but less autonomy as there will be institutional policies in place. In private practice, surgeons have autonomy over their schedule, staffing, and all decision making regarding the group. There tends to be higher earning potential in private practice but this potential is dependent on health care reimbursement. With these benefits comes the responsibility for all of the clinical, administrative, and financial duties of the office.

Location is another important consideration. Access to one's support system, lifestyle, and cost of living are aspects of location to consider. Depending on the type and scope of practice desired, location can also give a sense of what type of job opportunities will be available in certain areas. Academic centers will often times be found in urban, densely populated cities. In more rural areas, the practices may be smaller in size with mixed practice opportunities being more common. It may be prudent to cast a wider net if the applicant is open to location rather than starting with a narrow search as this will naturally broaden opportunities that one may have otherwise not considered.

Perhaps one of the most critical portions to consider for the first job is figuring out whether it has the infrastructure and staff to support one's goals and continued growth. What are the must-haves and what are aspects of the job that are more flexible? Why is the institution adding or looking for a new partner? Do they have the case volume to maintain and bolster one's skills? A lot of these answers will come later on in the search during the interview process.

Hand-in-hand with these considerations is culture and mentorship. The number of partners and their availability and willingness to guide and mentor a new graduate should be strongly considered. Understanding personally what type of mentorship would be beneficial at this stage is important to think on. Residents who are applying should set up a meeting with mentors to discuss these ideas. It provides an opportunity to get feedback, reflect, and get their own experiences with the process.

The Search

When considering the search for the right first job, the primary questions are when and where. Sterbling and colleagues[5] published survey results for board-certified cardiothoracic surgeons with regards to their first job. The optimal time to start searching and interviewing has been elusive. In this survey, 86.9% interviewed between October and March of final year. Around 79.7% signed contracts before completing training. Our recommended guideline would be to have the preparation phase as discussed earlier finalized by the conclusion of the second to last year, and to start searching and applying to jobs early to mid-year of the final year so that interviews are occurring around the middle of the year (**Table 3**).

There is not a single best resource to use for the job search. Available resources include the cardiothoracic community, national conferences, online employment sites, and recruiters. Perhaps one of the most useful is the small professional network. Program directors, division chair, and faculty often hear about opportunities from the people they know at various programs. Residents who are starting the job search should speak with their faculty, mentors and colleagues at other programs, and industry representatives. Another great opportunity is networking at annual meetings (AATS, STS). The STS meeting has a career fair, and often serves as a meeting place for practices and applicants. If feasible, it may be helpful to attend when possible but especially during the final year when interviewing. Alumni from applicant's respective programs (previous residents and fellows) or interview trail colleagues who are also interviewing are also good resources as they may have insight on places looking and can share their own interview experiences, and vice versa.

There are also various online employment sites with regularly updated job postings. These include CTSnet.org, Doximity.com, JAMA, NEJM, and Practicelink, to name a few. Recruiting agencies can also be helpful. Recruiters can be employed by a hospital or physician group for jobs that are or are not necessarily advertised online. They can tailor search criteria to jobs they have available and coordinate meetings and interviews.

During the search, if an applicant sees a listing for a job that he or she either does not quality for or that is missing a vital aspect of his or her must-haves, it is probably best to not apply to that job to save both parties time.

The Interview

There is no magic number of interviews to obtain, schedule, or complete. Residents should interview at places they are strongly considering based off the initial phone or virtual conversations. The Sterbling and colleagues[3] survey had a median of 4 interviews with a range of 3 to 6.

Once invited for an interview, preparation should be similar to that of past interviews. The applicant should research and learn as much as they can about the practice, institution, and community. Resources include the practice web site and the cardiothoracic surgery network. A schedule is usually provided with a list of the people that the applicant will meet. The candidate should learn about these people and have individualized and genuine questions prepared. Questions can include details about the practice, how many hospitals there are and which the new hire would practice at, case

Table 3
Recommended timeline of job search events during the final year of training

Last year of training[a]	Job Search Targets
July to September	Solidify priorities, goals, and characteristics of ideal job
	Begin exploring through various avenues
	Start applying
October to December	Phone interviews
	First visits/interviews
January to March	Second interview
	Consider offers
March to May	Negotiate contract details
	Begin state licensing process for accepted or high potential positions
May to July	Begin credentialing
	Relocate
July to September	Consider taking time between training/first job (typically 1 mo or less)
	Start your well-deserved first job as a cardiothoracic surgeon

[a] It is highly recommended that one establishes a reputation for being professional, industrious, courteous, and caring throughout training (and beyond).

From Macke RA, Ghanta R, Starnes S, Harken AH. So, you are looking for a job: Pearls for a successful first cardiothoracic job search. The Journal of Thoracic and Cardiovascular Surgery. 2018;156(4):1575-1584. doi:10.1016/j.jtcvs.2018.04.125; with permission.

volume and mix, teaching and research responsibilities, and culture and mentorship. If the opportunity arises, the applicant should take the time to interact with and ask questions to staff who work closely with the potential partners but who he or she may not necessarily have a formal interview with (eg, anesthesiologists, intensivists, perfusionists, administrative staff, nurses, advanced practice practitioners). These staff members can provide valuable insight on what it is like to work with the surgeons and team.

The interview experience will vary but will generally be one to two separate interview visits. The first interview visit will often be more than 2 days with a dinner with the surgeons. One of these days will likely consist of a full day of interviews with various members of the multidisciplinary team. There may be the opportunity to observe cases. Professional attire and conduct is a must. The candidate should listen intently to get an overview of the position, who he or she will work with, and resource allocation. The applicant should be kind and respectful to those he or she meets, maintain his or her level of enthusiasm throughout, and observe how people interact with one another. The applicant should also display confidence in his or her skillset and experiences thus far, and be able to highlight those qualities. For academic positions, it is important to be able to eloquently describe scholarly and research activities, and thoughtful future career goals.

After the first interview visit, it is useful to write down everything one remembers about the position, area, and people. The applicant should reflect and ask (1) can I see myself integrating well into the group, (2) will I have the support and mentorship needed to be successful (3) were there any questions that I want to follow-up with?

Not all programs have a second interview but it is fairly common. This visit often means that the candidate is in a small group of people the practice is seriously considering. That being said, the applicant should not go unless he or she is strongly considering the program as well. The applicant's significant other or partner may be invited to join during the second visit. This interview may involve faculty and staff that were missed meeting during the initial visit, and a realtor to look at housing options. During this visit, benefits and compensation may be discussed during or shortly after this visit. This second interview is a great time to ask any additional questions regarding clinical support, call responsibilities, expected operative and clinical days. It is a good idea to send personalized thank you emails after this visit. If the resident is strongly considering a position, asking his or her references to reach out to the program will further convey interest and can go a long way.

The Contract

Most employers will provide an offer letter or letter of intent. At this point, candidates realistically may still be interviewing or getting offers from multiple institutions, and may be weighing various options.

One should not sign a letter of intent if he or she is not seriously considering that specific practice. Similarly, if a program shows interest in the candidate, the candidate should respond in an expeditious manner. Both the applicant and potential employers are exploring their options but if serious interest is expressed on one or both sides, it is best to be upfront. Keep in mind that if an employer has made an offer, and the applicant wants to wait for other offers, that employer may very well move on to another applicant.

Formal contracts will often entail: compensation, benefits, responsibilities, terms and termination, and restrictive covenants. There may be many pages of detail, legal speak, and faculty codes. This aspect of finding the "right" first job will likely be the least familiar to the new graduate. We will provide an overview of the contract but it is often helpful to review the contract with a mentor, chair or program director, or an attorney.

Compensation will vary based on practice type. It can be guaranteed salary, purely productivity based, or a combination of the two. Most practices will offer a guaranteed salary start up period of two to 3 years. After the initial contract, most surgeons will transition to productivity, or relative value units (RVU) based. An RVU-based salary without any guaranteed salary start up period would be risky for the first job. The Association of American Medical Colleges and the Medical Group Management Association are great resources for evaluating salary. They provide published data on salary and work RVUs by region, academic rank, and expertise. These data are available for purchase but also may be available through the business or finance administrator of the applicant's current cardiothoracic surgery department.

Benefits will often be included in the contract as well. If not explicitly included, the applicant should inquire about the benefits package. Benefits include health and dental insurance, malpractice insurance, retirement plans, and paid leave. It also may include disability and life insurance, fringe benefits and relocation coverage. Benefits may vary widely from institution to institution, and may constitute an entire chapter. Be sure to understand the programs offered, vesting schedules, family coverage policies, childcare programs, and others. There are 2 major types of malpractice insurance, claims-made and occurrence based. The distinction between the 2 types is based on when you have coverage and when a claim is made. A claims-made policy covers incidents that occur when your policy is active. Both the incident and the claim must fall within the coverage period to be covered by insurance. With such policy, you may be able to add tail coverage that will protect you if a claim is filed after your coverage has ended. With occurrence-based malpractice insurance, the policyholder is covered for any incident while the policy was in place regardless of when the claim is made.

A section on responsibilities will be included in the contract. This will often review the scope of practice and call responsibility. For academic positions, the specific track (tenure vs nontenure) should be included. There should be some discussion about requirements for promotion, clinical and research expectations. It may highlight teaching or administrative duties as well. This is an important aspect of the contract to personally reflect and get feedback on regarding what track is the most realistic and aligned with one's goals.

Terms and termination are defined within the contract. The length of the initial employment and opportunities for partnership will be delineated. Reasons for termination, termination with or without cause, are often provided in detail. Termination for cause will often have notice with an opportunity for correction depending on the reasoning. Termination without cause means termination where either party can terminate without providing reasoning as long as there is sufficient notice. If the physician is terminating the contract within the startup period, there is often a payback requirement for the startup funding.

Restrictive covenants are an important component of the contract to understand. These are restrictions placed on the physician after they leave the institution. A covenant not to compete prohibits practice or competition within the same area. This will often specify a mile radius and time period for which this restriction is in place. A nonsolicitation covenant prohibits recruiting current patients or employees to his or her new practice. These clauses are often hard to negotiate on.

Once the applicant has a contract, it should be reviewed thoroughly, and reviewed with a trusted advisor or faculty. Another set of eyes will often bring up questions that the applicant may have otherwise not thought to ask. Once the candidate has a thoughtful set of questions or aspects of the contract that he or she may want to negotiate, a meeting should be set up with the finance administrator to discuss these aspects of the contract. He or she should negotiate aspects of the job that are important but also avoid exhaustive negotiation. Parts of the contract that practices may be more willing to consider are incentivized bonuses based on productivity, signing bonuses, student loan repayment, and start-up funds for projects.

When negotiating and considering a contract, the salary should often not be the most critical aspect of the job consideration. The applicant's level of confidence that he or she will be in a supportive, mentoring environment with the necessary components to succeed and grow should be. The practice may give a certain time period to sign the contract. The candidate should take that time to review the contract and any negotiated changes.

SUMMARY

There is no perfect or standardized "right" first job. It is all about preparing with the surrounding resources and community and finding the best fit. During the process of the job search and once the contract has been officially signed, one should take the time to reflect on all that has been accomplished.

DISCLOSURE

Dr N.A. Mokadam is a consultant for Medtronic, Abbott, SynCardia, Xylocor, and Carmat. Dr R. Kim has nothing to disclose with regard to commercial support.

REFERENCES

1. Mokadam NA. Pro Tips for Every CT Surgeon Searching for that First Job - Part I Preparation. STS Career Resources. https://www.sts.org/resources/career-resources/blog/pro-tips-every-ct-surgeon-searching-first-job-part-i. Accessed April 2023.

2. STS Workforce on Career Development. The Society of Thoracic Surgeons. https://www.sts.org/resources/career-resources. Accessed April 2023.

3. Mokadam NA. Pro Tips for Every CT Surgeon Searching for that First Job - Part II Interviews. STS Career Resources. https://www.sts.org/resources/career-resources/blog/pro-tips-every-ct-surgeon-searching-first-job-part-ii. Accessed April 2023.

4. Mokadam NA. Pro Tips for Every CT Surgeon Searching for that First Job - Part III Job Offer. STS Career Resources. https://www.sts.org/resources/career-resources/blog/pro-tips-every-ct-surgeon-searching-first-job-part-iii. Accessed April 2023.

5. Sterbling HM, Molena D, Rao SR, et al. Initial report on young cardiothoracic surgeons' first job: From searching to securing and the gaps in between. J Thorac Cardiovasc Surg 2019;158(2):632–41.e3.

6. Macke RA, Ghanta R, Starnes S, et al. So, you are looking for a job: Pearls for a successful first cardiothoracic job search. J Thorac Cardiovasc Surg 2018;156(4):1575–84.

Personal Finance Wellness for New Attendings

Russell Seth Martins, MD[a], Kostantinos Poulikidis, MD[a], Faiz Y. Bhora, MD[b],*

KEYWORDS

- Surgery • Finances • Investing • Retirement • Insurance

KEY POINTS

- It is crucial for new attending surgeons to be financially literate at an early stage in their professional careers, to ensure sound financial decision-making early on.
- It is highly advisable for surgeons to establish a financial team comprising of a financial advisor, attorney, and tax professional to assist with financial planning.
- Obtaining insurance for death, disability, illness, or injury is imperative for surgeons to create a safety net for a career in which they have invested significant time and resources.
- Retirement planning should commence early, with surgeons funding a retirement plan that may work under the broadest possible circumstances (ie, length of retirement, tax and market risk, and so forth).
- Although it may be tempting to indulge in personal life goals with newfound financial surplus, surgeons must exercise financial prudence and balance their lifestyle with their long-term financial obligations.

FINANCIAL MANAGEMENT AS A NEW ATTENDING

Surgeons are among the most highly educated health-care professionals, having invested much of their time and money into intensive education and training. However, a consequence of this lengthy training period, which may span on average 5 to 10 years after medical school,[1] is that surgeons reach their peak earning years later than nonphysicians and physicians from nonsurgical specialties. In addition, many surgeons carry hefty debts incurred during college and medical school. Thus, when surgeons finally take on practice as an attending, it is paramount that they learn to navigate this new financial landscape of their career.

However, this is easier said than done. Financial literacy is a glaring blind spot in medical education,[2] and therefore, surgeons are ill-equipped to manage personal finances. The first paycheck as a surgical attending is a considerable leap from a trainee's salary, and surgeons may tend to overspend their earnings. This behavior is also fueled by the notion that as a new attending one can finally reap the rewards of the often-touted delayed gratification of a medical career. Surgeons are perceived as having the highest income among specialist physicians,[3] and this is often a factor motivating students to pursue a surgical career.[4] Financial well-being is intricately linked to many aspects of an individual's personal and professional life, and achieving financial stability is key to leading a satisfying, happy, and productive life. In this article, we discuss strategies to help surgeons take control of their finances as they embark on one of the most exhilarating and challenging phases of their career.

[a] Division of Thoracic Surgery, Department of Surgery, Hackensack Meridian School of Medicine, Hackensack Meridian Health (HMH) Network, Edison, NJ 08820, USA; [b] Department of Surgery, Hackensack Meridian School of Medicine, Hackensack Meridian Health (HMH) Network, Edison, NJ 08820, USA
* Corresponding author. Hackensack Meridian Health (HMH) Network – Central Region, Hackensack Meridian School of Medicine, 65 James Street, Edison, NJ 08820.
E-mail address: faiz.bhora@hmhn.org

Thorac Surg Clin 34 (2024) 25–31
https://doi.org/10.1016/j.thorsurg.2023.08.002
1547-4127/24/© 2023 Published by Elsevier Inc.

BUILD A TEAM FOR FINANCIAL SUCCESS

The field of surgery is rife with the unexpected and the unknown, and surgeons typically like to feel in control of all aspects of their practice. However, just as successful surgical practice depends on multidisciplinary collaboration based on trust and diverse expertise, personal finance management is also best accomplished by the help of a team of qualified professionals. For surgeons at the start of their attending careers, this team should consist of a financial advisor and ideally, a tax professional and attorney(s) (eg, a contract attorney and estate attorney). Although hiring professionals to create a personal finance management team may seem to be an additional expense, the long-term value of a well-chosen team cannot be overstated.

The primary purpose of a financial advisor is to understand their clients' unique personal financial goals and help develop strategies to achieve them. In this regard, they educate clients regarding investment opportunities, monitor accounts to evaluate financial performance, and revise strategies for expected or unexpected life changes. Financial advisors may also serve as the "team lead" and can coordinate and liaison with other finance professionals on the team. When choosing a financial advisor, aim to select one who is a Certified Financial Planner who will act as a fiduciary and is bound to only provide advice that is in your best interest. In addition, it is important for surgeons to find an advisor with experience with the unique financial challenges and opportunities faced by those in the surgical profession. This can be achieved by exploring word-of-mouth recommendations from colleagues and superiors or by specifically inquiring about financial advisors with relevant experience at reputable asset management companies. Some surgical societies also offer recommendations to members regarding selection of finance professionals.[5] The cost of retaining a financial advisor varies widely and may have different payment structures such as commission based, fee based, or fee-only. With the fee-only structure, the advisor receives a fixed, annual fee based on a percentage (usually 0.5%–1.5%) of assets being managed. Fee-only advisors are generally seen as operating in a fiduciary capacity in that they have a legal and ethical obligation to act in their clients' best interests.

IMPROVE YOUR FINANCIAL LITERACY

The medical and surgical curricula impart a wide range of skills that enable surgeons to provide high-quality, complex, and multidisciplinary care to their patients. A surgeon's day-to-day job involves the ability to assimilate, synthesize, and simplify large amounts of information. These same skills provide a solid foundation to develop financial literacy. Surgeons are also the most risk averse among physicians,[6] which generally leads to safer financial decisions and investments. Thus, although surgeons possess the capacity to develop financial expertise, their hectic professional commitments may leave them pressed for time in which to do so. Nevertheless, surgeons must aim to consciously and gradually grow their financial literacy so that they can make better decisions and exercise more control over their personal finances.

There are a variety of easily accessible resources that can serve as an excellent starting point for financial self-education for surgeons. Books such as *The White Coat Investor* series,[7–9] *Financial Freedom Rx*,[10] *The Physician Philosopher's Guide to Personal Finance*,[11] and *The Physician's Guide to Personal Finance*[12] lay out financial principles in an easily digestible form for physicians. There are also many excellent personal finance management podcasts tailored for physicians, including "*The White Coat Investor Podcast*," "*The Freedom Formula for Physicians Podcast*," "*The Passive Income MD Podcast*," "*The Financial Residency Podcast*," and "*The Physician Philosopher Podcast*."[13] Surgeons may also consider subscribing to business and economics publications, such as the *Wall Street Journal*—although intended for an audience with a certain prerequisite level of financial savvy, these can provide valuable, technical, current insights into the financial world. Professional surgical societies, such as the American College of Surgeons,[14] also provide educational resources regarding personal finance management for surgeons. In addition to these resources, surgeons should not hesitate to seek the advice of financially stable senior attendings. The value of mentorship is recognized in all aspects of a physician's professional career and having a "money mentor" can help junior surgeons gain broader perspectives to help plan their financial futures. Financial advisors may also conduct routine educational sessions to bring their clients up to speed with current market trends. Finally, surgeons can learn a lot from engaging in active discussion with their financial advisors and can also apply some of their newly acquired knowledge to their current and future financial strategies. Moreover, given the potential to encounter conflicting advice from different self-education material, and the uniqueness of one's financial situation, it is best for young surgeons to consolidate and contextualize newly acquired information or advice with their trusted financial advisor.

GET INSURED

Surgeons thrive on predictability, and there are few things more satisfying to a surgeon than an operation that proceeds as expected. However, just as every surgeon must be prepared for the unpredictable in the operating room, it is also important for surgeons to equip themselves to combat any uncertainties in life. Understanding the importance of adequate insurance coverage is vital for surgeons in order to construct a safety net for a career in which they have invested significant time and resources. Surgeons must be insured against death, disability, illness or injury, medical malpractice, personal lawsuits, and destruction of property. In this article, we focus on life insurance and disability insurance.

Life insurance provides monetary support to one's dependents or beneficiaries in the event of one's passing away. This can enable the insured individual's family to maintain their lifestyle and continue with life plans. Life insurance can also be used to fulfill any outstanding financial obligations or debts, which may be particularly relevant during the early years of a surgeon's career. It is crucial to acquire adequate life insurance as early as possible, especially when one has dependents because the chosen policy is upheld regardless of any changes in health down the line and the costs are age-sensitive and health-sensitive (ie, more expensive the longer one waits). It is advisable to maintain life insurance equal to the present value of one's expected future earnings, with exact amounts varying according to one's dependents, existing finances, and time horizon. This philosophy is the basis of the Human Life Value theory, which guides the industry insurable limits of 30 times earnings while aged between 18 to 40 years, 20 times while in one's 40s, 15 times while in one's 50s, and then net worth-based thereafter. Employer-provided life insurance usually amounts to 2 times one's salary, with options to further increase coverage. It is important to thoroughly review the policies detailed in employer-provided life insurance packages, paying particular attention to the costs of carrying forward the same policy in case of a change of employer if the plan is portable. However, surgeons must also explore their options in purchasing their own life insurance plans independently to supplement employer-provided coverage. Consulting with one's financial advisor can help navigate the several options available.[15]

Disability insurance protects against loss of income in the event of a disability that prevents one from working. This may include chronic health conditions, injury, sensory problems, issues with mobility, and psychological disability.[16] Disability may be considered a "fate worse than death" because an uninsured surgeon who is unable to work because of disability is a greater financial burden on their family than if they passed away. Employer-provided disability insurance generally focuses on short-term disability. Long-term coverage usually amounts to a maximum of 50% to 60% of lost wages,[17] although some plans may cap out as low as US$5000 of monthly benefit (which may equate to roughly 10%–20% of income). Employer-provided disability insurance benefits are usually taxable and may have additional costs associated with carrying it forward when changing employers (if portable at all). In addition, it is also important to be cognizant of the definition of disability as per an employer-provided insurance plan, that is, if the operational definition is "any occupation" or "own occupation." Under the "any occupation" definition, a surgeon may not qualify for disability benefits if their disability leaves them with enough capability of working in an alternate capacity. However, the "own occupation" definition is more lenient and allows the policyholder to qualify for disability benefits if unable to work in their specific occupation. Thus, although employers do allow surgeons to voluntarily purchase increased coverage, it is important that surgeons consider independent disability insurance throughout their operative careers. Independent disability insurance plans must be specialty specific, with "own occupation" definitions, noncancellable, guaranteed renewable, and updateable as surgeons' income changes during the course of their career. These plans also usually have an option for cost-of-living adjustment, which increases benefits in accordance with inflation. Moreover, it is generally advisable to pay for independent disability insurance with after-tax income, so that the disability compensation received is not taxable. Disability insurances may be of 2 types, depending on the structure of premium payment. With a level premium disability insurance policy, participants pay a fixed premium at regular intervals for the duration of the term of the policy. However, a graded policy features lower premiums at the beginning of the term and increasingly higher premiums as the term progresses. A conversion from a graded policy to a level policy is possible. Choosing between the 2 depends on an estimation of the cumulative payments at the end of the term. Surgeons may consider making their independently purchased insurance their primary plan and treating their employer-provided insurance as a supplementary plan. Again, it is important to carefully review the terms and stipulations of an independently purchased plan with one's financial advisor.

Finally, umbrella insurance can provide additional liability protection beyond standard limits on homeowner, renter, automobile, or personal liability insurance. Umbrella insurance generally covers liability costs and legal fees involved in cases of bodily injury to others or damage to others' property. It is important to note that umbrella insurance does not usually cover medical malpractice or other forms of occupational liability because this insurance is usually provided by employers. Generally, umbrella insurance should at minimum equal to one's current net worth. The price of umbrella insurance varies according to risk associated with an individual's lifestyle, as higher risk invites greater liability.

LOANS AND DEBT

The average medical school graduate owes 7 times more than other college graduates. Medical school debt has almost quadrupled during the last 3 decades to an average of approximately US$224,000.[18] In addition, surgeons may have acquired additional loans for living expenses. Because carrying large debts can have a major negative influence on surgeons' financial and overall well-being, it is critical that surgeons prioritize and carefully plan debt-repayment strategies.

The terms "good debt" and "bad debt" are frequently used in discussion of loan acquisition and debt repayment. Generally, good debt is debt that holds the potential for long-term financial value by appreciation of asset value, income generation, or increasing earning potential. Examples include mortgages to purchase property, which has the potential to appreciate in value or student loans for college and medical school. Student loans are commonly paid back in installment amounts that are a fixed percentage of one's income. Given that an attending's salary is significantly higher than that of a trainee, attending surgeons must be prepared to pay back a greater gross amount than they were paying earlier. Another feature of good debt is that it has relatively lower interest rates. However, bad debt is considered detrimental to long-term financial well-being due to high interest rates, which may spiral out of control. Examples of bad debt include credit card debt, payday loans (short-term loans taken to cover unexpected expenses or bridge a gap in cash flow between paydays), and car loans.

A debt-repayment strategy should be carefully designed to suit one's personal financial situation. Generally, one should start by creating a budget for monthly income and expenses and determine what amount can be committed toward routine debt repayment. Next, this amount should be allocated to various debt obligations by creating a priority list. Generally, it is recommended that individuals should focus on clearing high-interest debts as early as possible (ie, the avalanche method) while continuing to make minimum payments on their low-interest debts. However, it may also be feasible to completely pay off smaller debts so that one can devote all future efforts toward paying off larger debts (ie, the snowball method). Credit card debt is typically high-interest and must be paid off regularly to avoid disastrous accumulation of compound interest. Surgeons should also be aware of medical school loan forgiveness opportunities that they can benefit from. The Public Service Loan Forgiveness is a public program that offers loan forgiveness to those working full time under qualifying employers (government organizations and certain tax-exempt nonprofit organizations) while making 120 qualifying loan payments (typically made monthly during a minimum period of 10 years). Finally, surgeons should consider using monetary windfalls (such as signing bonuses, work bonuses, or tax refunds) to pay back their debts and be cautious of incurring new debt while still paying off old loans.

PLANNING FOR RETIREMENT

Although it may seem counterintuitive or unnatural for new attending surgeons to begin to think about their retirement, there is no better time to begin than the present. Retirement planning begins with carefully determining one's expenses postretirement and using these to calculate an approximate annual budget.

Individual retirement arrangements (IRAs) are a form of personal savings that provide tax advantages for retirement savings. There are several different types of IRA,[19] such as the traditional IRA and Roth IRAs. Although there are no income limits for contributing to a traditional IRA, tax deductibility of contributions is limited for surgeons participating in an employer-sponsored plan and whose annual income exceeds the maximum limit (US$83,000 if filing single or US$136,000 if jointly). Roth IRAs source after-tax income but qualified withdrawals after retirement are accessible tax-free. Although contributing to a Roth IRA is not an option for most surgical attendings because of their modified adjusted gross income exceeding the annual limit, a backdoor Roth IRA offers the opportunity to take advantage of the benefit of the plan. To set up a backdoor Roth IRA, one can make after-tax contributions to a traditional IRA and complete a Roth conversion to port the funds into a Roth IRA. In 2023, the maximum annual contribution to a Roth IRA is US$6500 (or US$7500 if aged older than 50 years) annually.

Surgeons may also choose to partake in employer-sponsored retirement plans, among which options include:

- *401(k)*: A 401(k) plan allows employees to contribute a proportion of their income to their account. It also allows employers to contribute to employees' accounts, which may be done in the form of a dollar-for-dollar or percentage match. In the traditional (non-Roth) structure, the contributions to the 401(k) are made pretax (ie, excluded from the employee's taxable income) but the funds (including earnings) are taxable at retirement. For 2023, the annual contribution limit to a one-participant 401(k) plan is US$22,500 (with employer nonelective contributions up to 25% of compensation).[20] Roth contributions are commonly allowed in employer-provided 401(k) plans, and these are not subject to income limits like the Roth IRA.
- *403(b)*: A 403(b) plan is similar to a 401(k) plan and can be thought of as its counterpart that is offered by nonprofit organizations, tax exempt organizations, or government employers. For 2023, the annual contribution limit to a one-participant 403(b) plan is US$22,500.[21]
- *457(b)*: A 457(b) plan is employer-sponsored and sources pretax contributions from one's paycheck in addition to contributions to a 401(k)/403(b). Earnings on the retirement funds are also tax deferred. The 2 types of 457(b) plans are governmental and nongovernmental plans. In a governmental plan, savings are protected by a trust and can be carried into other accounts such as a 401(k)/403(b). In a nongovernmental plan, funds are subject to an employer's creditors and are not protected. For 2023, the annual contribution limit to a one-participant 457(b) plan is US$22,500.[22]
- *Health Savings Accounts (HSA)*: An HSA is a tax-advantaged personal savings account available to individuals with a high-deductible health plan (HDHP) to help save and pay for qualified medical expenses. To be eligible, the individual cannot be enrolled in any non-HDHP health insurance plan.

Contributions within an HSA can be invested in a variety of assets and can be carried forward each year. The funds within the HSA may be withdrawn tax-free to pay for qualified medical expenses. The funds may also be withdrawn to be used for reasons other than qualified medical expenses. In this case, one would have to pay taxes on this money and possibly a 20% penalty if the money is withdrawn before the individual is aged 65 years. In 2023, the maximum annual contribution to an HSA is US$3850.

Although surgeons should aim to maximize their contributions to tax-advantaged retirement savings accounts, it is also important to invest in other assets. Generally, it is advisable to diversify investments to reduce risks (not putting all eggs in one basket) and increase reward, with the investment strategy depending on an individual surgeon's risk tolerance, investment goals, and time to retirement. A diverse investment portfolio consists of a variety of different assets, including bonds, real estate, and stocks, across a variety of different businesses, sectors, and geographic regions. Again, consulting with one's financial advisor is the best way to chart out a personalized investment strategy to meet one's goals.

LIFESTYLE AND FAMILY

Beginning practice as a new surgical attending can be the first experience of significant financial surplus for surgeons. It may be tempting to immediately leap into fulfilling long-awaited personal life goals, such as buying a house or car, getting married, having kids, or traveling. However, it is important for surgeons to exercise financial caution and recognize their long-term financial responsibilities to themselves and their families. Hitting the sweet spot between spending and saving requires careful strategizing, planning, and reflection.

This process should begin with constructing a comprehensive, long-term plan that describes specific life goals and financial targets with the approximate monetary amounts required and approximate timelines. Getting married involves several financial considerations and surgeons contemplating marriage should discuss joint finances, income and debt levels, tax implications, and insurance coverage with their prospective partners before tying the knot. Family planning also requires financial thought and due attention must be paid to matters such as health insurance for children, paid maternity and paternity leave, and childcare expenses. This is also an important time to review and adjust life and disability insurance to ensure adequate financial protection for one's family. In addition, if one wishes to contribute toward their child's future education, it is important to start saving as early as possible. This begins with determining a target amount and reviewing the various savings plans that are available, such as a 529 or a custodial account. A 529 is a tax-advantaged savings plan that is usually sponsored by a state or an educational institution. It allows funds to be invested and grow tax-free provided that they are used for qualified educational expenses (typically for higher education; certain states may also allow 529 funds to be used tax-free for K-12 tuition). Some states may also offer a tax deduction or credit for contributions to a 529 education savings plan. A custodial savings account is managed by a custodian until the beneficiary reaches the age of maturity (18 or 21 years old depending on the state), with the funds being available for educational expenses. However, since the funds are counted as assets of the beneficiary, they may influence financial aid eligibility.

Buying a house may be an important personal and financial landmark for surgeons, and it is important to invest serious efforts into the decision-making process. The first step is to determine the need to buy a house given the local housing market and one's mid-term to long-term career plans. If buying a house is in one's best interest, individuals must begin by carefully calculating a budget. Factors to be considered include income, expenses, financial goals, and house-associated costs such as property taxes, homeowner's insurance, and maintenance. When exploring mortgages, it is important to take advantage of physician-specific options that may be available. A physician's loan is available for licensed medical professionals who are still paying off student loans. These mortgage products may feature a lower down payment than traditional mortgages, relaxed lending standards, higher debt-to-income ratio allowance, lower interest rates, and no private mortgage insurance requirements.

Finally, it is also important for young surgeons to maintain a reasonable degree of liquidity of their funds because these can help cover emergency expenses and periods of job transition. In addition, liquidity may also enable young surgeons to remain flexible and better capitalize on opportunities for personal and professional growth.

SUMMARY

Managing personal finances is an essential skill for surgeons, particularly those beginning their careers as attendings. The high income earned as a surgical attending may be a double-edged sword because it can lead to poor financial habits such as overspending. Moreover, due to their busy schedules, surgeons may find themselves hard pressed for time to increase their financial literacy and manage personal finances. It is paramount that one focuses on building a financial team, which includes a financial advisor, to help strategize budgeting, investing, and retirement planning. Additionally, there are a variety of easily accessible resources that surgeons can use for self-education regarding personal financial management. By staying disciplined with spending and investing habits, surgeons can not only achieve their financial goals but also enjoy greater peace of mind, success, and fulfillment in their personal and professional lives.

DECLARATIONS
Conflicts of Interest

None.

Funding

None.

Ethics Approval

None required.

ACKNOWLEDGMENTS

The authors would like to thank Bryan M. Kuderna, CFP (Certified Financial Planner), MSFS (Master of Science in Financial Services), RICP (Retirement Income Certified Professional), LUTCF (Life Underwriter Training Council Fellow) for reviewing this article and offering insight and suggestions.

DISCLOSURE

The authors have nothing to disclose.

REFERENCES

1. Jeekel J. Crucial times for general surgery. Ann Surg 1999;230(6):739–41. Epub 2000/01/01.
2. Jayakumar KL, Larkin DJ, Ginzberg S, et al. Personal financial literacy among US medical students. MedEdPublish 2017;6(35):35.
3. Puertas EB, Orellana RA, Muñoz BE, et al. Factors influencing the choice of a career in primary care among medical students in Central America. Rev Panam Salud Publica 2020;44:e94–.
4. Zaheer F, Rehman HU, Fareed W, et al. Factors Affecting the Choice of a Career in the Field of Surgery Among Medical Students of Karachi. Cureus 2018;10(11):e3542. Epub 2019/01/17.

5. New York Chapter American College of Surgeons Selects Altfest as its Preferred Wealth Management Education Provider. New York Chapter American College of Surgeons; 2010 3rd May 2023; Available at: https://www.altfest.com/ny-acs/.

6. Pikkel D, Pikkel Igal YS, Sharabi-Nov A, et al. Are doctors risk takers? Risk Manag Healthc Pol 2016; 9:129–33. Epub 2016/07/07.

7. Dahle JM, Bernstein WJ. The white coat investor: a doctor's guide to personal finance and investing. White Coat Investor, LLC; 2014.

8. James M. Dahle JC. The White Coat Investor's Financial Boot Camp: A 12-Step High-Yield Guide to Bring Your Finances Up to Speed. 2019.

9. Dahle JM. The White Coat Investor's Guide to Asset Protection: How to Protect Your Life Savings from Frivolous Lawsuits and Runaway Judgments. 2022.

10. Chirag P. Shah JS. Financial Freedom Rx: The Physician's Guide to Achieving Financial Independence. 2021.

11. Turner JD. The Physician Philosopher's Guide to Personal Finance: The 20% of Personal Finance Doctors Need to Know to Get 80% of the Results. 2019.

12. Steiner J. The Physician's Guide to Personal Finance: The review book for the class you never had in medical school. 2013.

13. Farhat C. 7 Personal Finance Podcasts for Doctors. 2022; Available from: https://www.elfi.com/personal-finance-podcasts-for-doctors/.

14. Surgeons ACo. Personal Financial Wellness Resources. 2020 1st May 2023; Available at: https://www.facs.org/for-medical-professionals/practice-management/financial-wellness/.

15. Danise A. Types Of Life Insurance Policies. 2023 1st May 2023; Available at: https://www.forbes.com/advisor/life-insurance/types/.

16. Nouri Z, Dill MJ, Conrad SS, et al. Estimated Prevalence of US Physicians With Disabilities. JAMA Netw Open 2021;4(3):e211254–.

17. Monaco K. Disability insurance plans: trends in employee access and employer costs. 2015 3rd May 2023; Available from: https://www.bls.gov/opub/btn/volume-4/disability-insurance-plans.htm.

18. Hanson M. Average Medical School Debt. 2022 2nd May 2023; Available at: https://educationdata.org/average-medical-school-debt.

19. Service IR. Individual Retirement Arrangements (IRAs). cited 1st May 2023; Available at: https://www.irs.gov/retirement-plans/individual-retirement-arrangements-iras.

20. Service IR. 401(k) Plans. (1st May 2023); Available from: https://www.irs.gov/retirement-plans/401k-plans.

21. Service IR. IRC 403(b) Tax-Sheltered Annuity Plans. 1st May 2023; Available from: https://www.irs.gov/retirement-plans/irc-403b-tax-sheltered-annuity-plans.

22. Service IR. IRC 457(b) Deferred Compensation Plans. 1st May 2023; Available from: https://www.irs.gov/retirement-plans/irc-457b-deferred-compensation-plans.

The Growing Years
Promoting Yourself in the First 5 Years

Kirsten A. Freeman, MD

KEYWORDS

- Transition to practice • Networking • Early career surgeon

KEY POINTS

- The first 5 years in practice are ones of exponential growth.
- Transitioning from training to surgical practice can be broken down into clinical growth, professional growth, and personal growth.
- Promoting yourself during those first 5 years is crucial for your future.

INTRODUCTION

Postgraduate medical training can be a long and arduous road, particularly for those in the surgical subspecialties. After medical school, many require close to a decade to complete residency and fellowship. A residency and fellowship certificate does not quite embody the literal blood, sweat, and tears that goes into those years. The piece of paper is analogous to an attendance record: dates, location, and type of training. That general surgery certificate does not show the gumption it takes to stand up in front of an audience of residents and attending surgeons to present a mortality at a conference, it does not show the grit it takes to make the phone call to an attending in the middle of the night, it does not show the mentorship of junior residents and medical students, the lost nights of sleep, the missed events, the falling asleep with a face in a book. No, that certificate does not quite do those years justice.

The fellowship years, although shorter, are packed with an exponential level of difficulty that is hard to truly comprehend. With this change came an exponential increase in excitement but also stress. However, by this time, you were a professional resident. For many people that went through the traditional training route for cardiothoracic surgery it involved 5 years of general surgery, 2 years of research, and 2 to 3 years of fellowship.

After 10 years of graduate medical education, the role is well-known and the script easy to follow. Clinically, you see a consult, make decisions, and call your attending to see if they agree. Professionally, you find your surgical societies—sign up as a resident member, look for resident opportunities on the website, and when the annual meeting comes up be sure to note resident-specific items. As a trainee, the graduate medical education emails target you with leadership opportunities. Your department may have research laboratories with a lineage of hosting residents in the research years longer than you have been alive. Moreover, every attending has the potential to be a mentor, whether it be a surgical mentor, research mentor, educational mentor, or a personal mentor.

It is often said that the real learning comes in the first 5 years of your surgical practice after training is complete. There are several transitions that must be made to define your new role as an attending surgeon. Establishing these transitions can be difficult but trying to promote yourself while undergoing these awkward transitions can be taxing but crucial. Whether you are in private practice trying to obtain referrals to build your practice or in an academic setting where you are trying to find your niche, promoting yourself along the way is imperative for your future growth. There are 3 core transitions in the first 5 years: (1) clinical, (2) professional, and (3) personal (**Fig. 1**).

Department of Surgery, Division of Cardiovascular Surgery, University of Florida, PO Box 100129, Gainesville, FL 32610-0129, USA
E-mail address: Kirsten.freeman@surgery.ufl.edu

Thorac Surg Clin 34 (2024) 33–38
https://doi.org/10.1016/j.thorsurg.2023.08.003
1547-4127/24/© 2023 Elsevier Inc. All rights reserved.

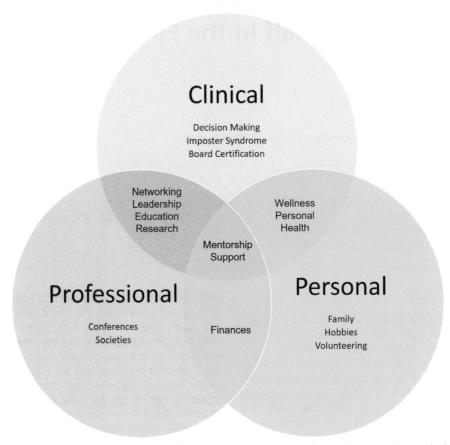

Fig. 1. Venn diagram showing the 3 core transitions of clinical, professional, and personal growth during your first 5 years in practice.

CLINICAL TRANSITIONS

After completion of surgical training, you have a certificate that states you have completed the necessary time and caseload to practice. You have signed a contract and been given privileges to perform surgery. Just put on your scrubs and go operate, right?

Transitioning from Trainee/Decision-Making

Decision-making in surgery is something learned from years' worth of exposures to complex medical and surgical problems aligned with textbook learning, examinations, mentors, consensus guidelines, and so forth. As a resident, there was always another person at the other end of the phone or across the operating room table to explicitly or implicitly agree with you in your decision-making. Losing the explicit agreement when you transition to an attending was expected. However, when an attending was scrubbed in but did not say anything it was still feedback. It implied you were doing the right thing as a resident, and it was ok to keep going. That loss of a mentor in the

operating room can make each step of the operation feel longer and fraught with more decisions. The more decisions you make, the more comfortable you will be making the decision the next time but understanding your limitations and knowing when to call for help is just as important. *Promoting yourself in the surgical arena means being a safe and competent surgeon, and knowing your limitations is paramount to that success.* Although you are managing your successes and failures in the operating room, you must also determine your referral base and familiarize yourself with key partners to work toward a successful surgical practice. Additionally, meeting with your coders and billers is extremely advantageous in understanding required documentation. All these in combination will contribute to clinical success.

Managing Failure/Imposter Syndrome

When you find yourself in a situation where you have reached your limit of knowledge or surgical ability, calling for help may feel like a failure. *Aligning yourself with surgical mentors is part of the process to reach your full potential as a surgeon.*[1] Imposter syndrome, the feeling of anxiety, self-doubt, and incompetence despite external evidence supporting competence and high-level performance are common among new surgical attendings.[2] There will be small bumps and large bumps along the way early in a surgical career but allying yourself with other early career surgeons can help support your progress during the transition out of training. These other early career surgeons may be people you trained with, met at a conference or a training course, or crossed paths with during the interviewing process. They can be in your own specialty or in another specialty. They then become part of your network of allies during your career as you both move into more senior years.

Certification

Operating independently and safely is a crucial step in your progress as a new attending surgeon. Unfortunately, that is not all it takes to continue on in your early career. Board certification is a crucial step in the surgical transition, and passing the board examination is not a foregone conclusion. Written board examination pass rate was 85% in 2021 and oral board pass rate was 75% and 85% for the 2 separate 2021 examinations.[3] Developing a study plan and being disciplined to comply with your plan is key. Unfortunately failing is a legitimate possibility, and many excellent surgeons have failed the examination. If retaking the examination, reach out to others to assess your study plan and maintain a support network throughout the process. *When your board certification is obtained, share the success with mentors, educators, friends, family, and employers as it is not only your achievement but also one for all of those who have helped you along the way.* Board certification is a crucial step in your professional career and a hurdle that must be surpassed to promote yourself.

PROFESSIONAL TRANSITIONS

Operating and achieving desired outcomes are essential parts of a surgeon's career. There are, however, additional obligations to the surgical profession. *Education, leadership, mentorship, research, and networking are pillars that contribute to the future of the field and are fundamentals for advancing and promoting your career.*

Education and Mentorship

When taking the Hippocratic Oath as physicians we cited "to teach them this art, if they shall want to learn it."[4] There are droves of undergraduate students and medical students across the nation interested in a career in surgery that would give up their free time to shadow a surgeon in the operating room. An afternoon in the operating room may be all it takes to inspire the next generation of surgeons.[5] Taking on teaching responsibilities, however, is often at odds with surgical efficiency or may take away time from other valuable work or your personal time. *When a teaching or mentorship opportunity arises, first you must determine if it is an obligation or an opportunity.* Obligations would be considered part of your contract, that is, if a residency training program exists and a resident is part of your case you are, by definition, an educator. Educators come in all forms. You may be an educator where the resident simply learns from watching and listening to your decision-making, or you may be an educator where you actively participate with preoperative, intraoperative, and postoperative direct teaching where you provide the opportunity to operate, to ask questions during the process, provide guidance, and then ultimately give feedback. As a medical student if you felt like you had good rapport with a resident or attending that gave you positive verbal feedback, you would reach out to them for an evaluation for that rotation. Similarly, if you were given positive verbal feedback from a trainee or mentee, it is helpful to keep them in mind as a resource if you require an evaluation.

Additionally, there are many teaching and mentorship opportunities that may cross your desk. Moreover, if you have a passion for education, you will find that these opportunities start to multiply. If education and mentorship are part of your purpose, then reach out to the surgery clerkship director and volunteer your services. Identify people on the medical school admissions committee and ask how to be involved with applicants and the interview process. Email the anatomy professor and ask to be involved in dissections or lectures. Look out for emails about local science fairs asking for judges. There are hundreds of opportunities waiting for teaching and mentoring the next generation. Each time you participate in an event, note the date and organization for tracking purposes. Email your leadership with pictures of the event and give them feedback about whether it was worthwhile. This will serve a dual purpose to both let them know about the event in general, and your participation in the event. Your feedback will function to aid in recommending, or not, that event to other faculty in the future.

Leadership

Leadership is paramount in surgery as the surgeon is leading the orchestra in the operating room.

Building both your leadership in and out of the operating room as a junior attending in the first 5 years of practice can be a challenge, and it depends on many factors. Leadership in the operating room can be affected by a multitude of elements, including but not limited to the seniority of the staff, staff burnout, location of practice, and so forth. It also can be affected by gender, age, or race of surgeon.[6] Imposter syndrome can weigh heavily on your ability to be a leader in the operating room but over time as you build days into months into years of practice, the leadership in the operating room often comes naturally. Leadership opportunities in the hospital and on campus, however, may not come as easily, and often require seeking out the opportunities and even creating your own.

In a large university setting, there are multiple levels of leadership opportunities. Start by looking within your division, then expand to the department, college of medicine, and university. There is a need to address wellness in medicine,[7] and if your division does not have a wellness director then ask if you can start a program. Similarly, there is a critical need for diversity, equity, and inclusion (DEI) in cardiothoracic surgery.[8,9] There are not only leadership opportunities in championing wellness and DEI but also a fundamental importance to patient care in advancing these matters in our field. In a private and academic setting, contact your leadership teams and seek their support for starting these programs.

Involve yourself with faculty search committees, graduate medical educational committees, residency interview committees, and so forth. There are hundreds of emails that cross your desk with leadership opportunities. These committees are chances to get more involved but are also networking opportunities for junior faculty members and can be a springboard for future or more substantial commitment. Again, it is important to share your involvement with your own division chief and department chair so that they not only know your contribution but so know where their faculty member's time is being spent. They may even seek you out if they want further information on that topic or ask you to present on the topic at a faculty meeting or grand rounds.

Research

Mentorship is a common theme for a junior faculty member but in the realm of research, it continues to be vital to your success. Even if you already have a PhD and wish to continue your work on a specific topic, you will still require assistance and knowledge from those around you who can aid in your search for laboratory space, personnel, and logistics at your institution. A research mentor may happen naturally as your interests become affiliated with a more senior researcher, or you may find yourself cold emailing someone within your interested field. Either way, as your curiosity increases in a topic, you should reach out to your division chief and ask if they have contacts that work in that field. Additionally, as you volunteer for committees and events, you may find that it takes you into a realm that you had not previously considered for your research because you are further exposed to what your local affiliation has to offer.

If you do not have a robust research background and are starting from scratch, it is best to *start with writing up your research. Begin with case reports, retrospective reviews, and small case series and submit to your local, regional, and then national conferences.* Furthermore, signing up to review articles not only expands your knowledge base but exposes you to the cutting edge of new research and gives you the opportunity to understand what information is important in research and what topics interest you. Reviewing articles is also an important step toward being considered an expert in your field. The more articles you review, and the timelier they are completed, the more your name will be associated with that topic.

Networking

Cardiothoracic surgery is a relatively small field in medicine, and the American Board of Thoracic Surgery notes that almost 9200 certificates have been issued since its formation in 1948.[10] With less than 10,000 practicing thoracic surgeons in the United States, you not only can meet the giants in our field but also work alongside them just by seeking out opportunities that are already within your reach. Networking is extremely valuable early in your career for innumerable reasons. Networking starts with simply signing up for your local, state, regional, and national organizations. Thoracic Surgery Directors Association,[11] CTSNet,[12] and Women in Thoracic Surgery[13] all have a compilation of regional, national, and international organizations easily accessible on their websites. Selection of which organizations to join depends on your location, current, and future interests. There also innumerable other organizations not exclusive to thoracic surgeons that you may join including the American College of Surgeons, the American Heart Association, and so forth.

In order to find your local and statewide organizations, you should talk with your colleagues and search online to find your resources. Your job may even reimburse you for some or all the membership fees, depending on the number of organizations you join. Remember, however, membership fees go up as an attending and you may have a financial limitation in signing up for all available organizations. Signing up for your local and/or statewide organization is a great way to meet the surgeons you will work with closely during your career. You may be accepting transfers from them or sending transfers to them, and obtaining their contact information may streamline the pipeline and allow for more readily accessible transfer of data. Additionally, local/state conferences are an excellent pathway for submitting posters, obtaining podium presentations, and establishing a presence on committees as a junior attending. Moreover, if there is not a robust organization locally or statewide, you can be instrumental in establishing one.

As you work toward obtaining a local presence, continue to be involved regionally and nationally as the prospects unfold. Once you are on the email listserv for regional and national organizations, you will note many meaningful ways to become more involved. *Imposter syndrome may prevent you from applying for positions, as you may not feel like you are an expert yet.* Do not let being a junior faculty member prevent you from participation in local, regional, and even national committees. You have completed rigorous training and your perspective as a recent graduate is indispensable on committees. Being on a regional or national committee will allow you to meet other surgeons with similar interests and have even more purpose when attending the conferences.

There are many facets to attending conferences. Setting up your weekend to address your interests is paramount, and you must have goals in mind before attending the conference including who you want to meet. (Dafflisio G, Abdelrehim A, Han J, Nguyen T. Attending your first academic cardiothoracic conference: Comprehensive guide for trainees and students. Submitted to J Thorac Cardiovasc Surg April 2023, under review). Although it may be easier to introduce yourself to another attending surgeon once you are an attending surgeon yourself, meeting a stranger can still be uncomfortable. It is notable to remember that it will likely take several meetings before someone remembers you. Being succinct but informative in your brief introduction including your name, type of surgery you perform, practice type, and location will help when you both introduce and reintroduce yourself. If you have met them previously, including any online event, note that in your introduction as a reference to an earlier meeting. Networking is simply adding people to your initially small circle of colleagues. As you add more people to your circle, it becomes an interwoven web with a vast reach. All it takes is reaching out your hand and introducing yourself.

Finally in networking, social media must be addressed. There are many social media platforms that each has a different purpose in networking. Facebook, Instagram, and Twitter are the most highly used networks currently. You must adhere to the rules of your institution and patient privacy laws while you are sharing information online. Rules regarding online engagement are both simple and complex for a young faculty member. *If you want to engage an audience on a social network, then post events and topics that are meaningful to you.* However, there must also be a warning with social media. Posting controversial topics may have consequences for your job and reputation, and therefore, you must always consider the influence of anything that you put online. Additionally, highlighting both successes and failures is also beneficial if you also have mentees as social media followers, so they can see that strife is normal. Social media is an incredible networking tool where you can follow hundreds or thousands of people without having to be in the same room. You can interact with their posts and ask questions. You can promote your own work, your institution, your mentors, and your mentees. Most importantly, you can connect with people that will be lifelong colleagues, resources, and mentors.

PERSONAL TRANSITIONS

For decades, there has been a countdown and a plan for "what's next." Finish undergraduate degree and apply for medical school. Complete medical school and apply for residency. Finish residency and apply for fellowship. Finish fellowship and start practice. Every resident or fellow has a countdown to graduation. Now that you are in your first job out of training, it seems too far off to have a countdown to retirement, so now what? The focus is no longer on what is next but what is happening now. *Cultivating your relationships, your hobbies, your finances, and your health are important steps into the personal transition that comes with the first 5 years in practice.* Nurturing your support network (that may have taken a backseat during training) is fundamental to the encouragement you will need to navigate through failures and celebrate your successes. Additionally, managing your finances including life insurance, disability insurance, savings plans, and debt payments are an important part of your growth as a junior attending. Do not be afraid to ask colleagues for help navigating through your first home purchase or finding help with taxes. Furthermore, sign up for that long overdue dental appointment and meet with a primary care physician. Maintain your own well-being so you can be a healthy surgeon for your own patients.

Finally, take the additional time you may have found and give back. You may have a higher salary and are able to financially contribute to charity but now you also have more time. Your time is just as valuable as your donations. Most people go into medicine because they want to help. Dedicating just a few hours to volunteer work provides a renewal of the mission you set out to achieve when you started medical school.

SUMMARY

When you walk into your first day as a newly minted surgeon, understanding the transitions you will go through can help alleviate some of the stress. Day by day, obstacle by obstacle, you will grow into your role. Your support network of mentors and other new surgeons will help you achieve clinical success and fight imposter syndrome. Clinically, professionally, and personally you will grow more in the first years after training than many other years in your life.

Promoting yourself clinically revolves around being a competent surgeon. Specifically, knowing when to call for help is of utmost importance early in your career. Familiarizing yourself with and getting to know your referral base is essential to building a practice, and completing your board certification fulfills a clinical obligation. Professionally, you will need to work with your partners, mentors, and colleagues to realize your goals in leadership, research, and education. Additionally, share your successes, not only to promote yourself but also to contribute to the overall success of your group, division, department, and university. Finally, networking early in your career provides an avenue for future collaboration, and attendance at conferences, membership in professional societies, and usage of social media can contribute to successfully navigating meeting new colleagues. The first 5 years are a daunting transition but with assistance from your support network, you can thrive.

ACKNOWLEDGMENTS

The author would like to acknowledge University of Florida, UF Health Shands, the Department of Surgery, Division of Cardiovascular Surgery for their support in my transition to practice. I would also like to thank my mentors, colleagues, friends, and family who also supported my training and transition to practice.

DISCLOSURES

The author has no conflict of interest and no financial disclosure.

REFERENCES

1. Odell D, Edwards M, Fuller S, et al. The art and science of mentorship in cardiothoracic surgery: A systemic review of the literature. Ann Thorac Surg 2022; 133(4):1093–100.
2. Sarosi G, Klingensmith M. Entrustable professional activities, a tool for addressing sex bias and the imposter syndrome? Ann Surg 2022;275(2):230–1.
3. American Board of Surgery Report to the Thoracic Surgery Directors Association, at https://tsda.org/wp-content/uploads/2022/06/ABTS-Report-to-TSDA-6-2-2022.pdf. Accessed May 1, 2023.
4. National Institute of Health, National Library of Medicine: Hippocratic Oath, at https://www.nlm.nih.gov/hmd/greek/greek_oath.html#:~:text=The%20Hippocratic%20Oath%20(%CE%9F%CF%81%CE%BA%CE%BF%CF%82)%20is,number%20of%20professional%20ethical%20standards. Accessed May 1, 2023.
5. Brennan J, Purlee M, Sharaf O, et al. Never too early: the impact of a shadowing programme in paediatric and congenital cardiac surgery for undergraduate college students. Cardiol Young 2023;33(4):514–9.
6. Parikh P, Kipfer S, Crawford T, et al. Unmasking bias and perception of lead surgeons in the operating room: A simulation based study. Am J Surg 2022; 223(1):58–63.
7. Fajardo R, Vaporciyan A, Starnes S, et al. Implementation of wellness into a cardiothoracic training program: A checklist for a wellness policy. J Thorac Cardiovasc Surg 2021;161(6):1979–86.
8. Godoy L, Hill E, Cooke D. Social Disparities in Thoracic Surgery Education. Thorac Surg Clin 2022;32(1):91–102.
9. Cooke D, Godoy L, Preventza O, et al. The importance of a diverse specialty: Introducing the STS workforce on diversity and inclusion. Ann Thorac Surg 2019;108(4):1000–5.
10. American Board of Thoracic Surgery Available at: https://www.abts.org/. Accessed May 1, 2023.
11. Thoracic Surgery Directors Association: Resources Available at: https://tsda.org/resources/related-links/. Accessed May 1, 2023.
12. CTSNet: Organizations Available at: https://www.ctsnet.org/organizations. Accessed May 1, 2023.
13. Women in Thoracic Surgery: Organizations Available at: https://wtsnet.org/career-resources/ct-surgical-organizations/. Accessed May 1, 2023.

Becoming a Cardiothoracic Surgical Educator

Amelia W. Wong, DO[a], Taryne A. Imai, MD, MEHP[b],*

KEYWORDS

- Surgeon educator • Surgical education • Scholarship and scholarly activity • Educational portfolio
- Faculty development

KEY POINTS

- In the current era of cardiothoracic training, the role of the educator is integral in ensuring that training is equitable for all levels of learners.
- Scholarship is the fundamental factor that distinguishes an educator from a teacher.
- Surgical educators need to be more than content experts and must acquire a variety of relevant knowledge domains to be an effective educator.
- Many educational activities are not captured by the traditional curriculum vitae, and therefore, educators' contributions to their institutions may be better displayed with an educational portfolio to appropriately demonstrate their scholarly work.
- The surgical educator academic track is different from a surgical scientist track in terms of skills, work performed, documentation, and promotion requirements.

INTRODUCTION

The current era in cardiothoracic training is changing rapidly and is a completely different teaching environment than before. With integrated 6-year and 4 + 3 programs increasing in numbers every year, the cardiothoracic surgery educator must now expand their teaching practices. In addition to training traditional cardiothoracic surgery residents who have completed a general surgery residency, the cardiothoracic surgery educator must now be able to teach medical students, interns, residents of all postgraduate years, and fellows obtaining specialty training. More than ever, the role of the educator is integral in ensuring that curricula, instructional strategies, and assessment are tailored to ensure that training is equitable for all levels of learners.

THE CLINICIAN-EDUCATOR

The "clinician-educator" is a term referring to a physician whose primary role is caring for patients and who has formally incorporated educational principles and scholarship.[1] The concept of the clinician-educator likely began in the 1980's when medical education was undergoing major changes as patient care moved from the inpatient to the ambulatory setting. The role of the clinician-educator developed as a means to fill the teaching gap for residents and medical students in ambulatory settings. Therefore, the early clinician-educators were often primary care physicians who brought pedagogy and curricular design into medical schools.[2] They included patients in their teaching and differentiated themselves from other clinicians by using evidence-based educational constructs to teach around patient illness and wellness. Early clinician-educators eventually converted those constructs and innovative teaching techniques into scholarship.

The definition of the clinician-educator has evolved over time and has become broader and more inclusive. Clinician-educators now encompass a diverse group of health care professionals, including not only physicians and surgeons of all specialties but also those who are not physicians.

[a] Department of Surgery, Queen's University Health System / University of Hawaii, Honolulu, Hawaii;
[b] Thoracic Surgery, Department of Surgery, Queen's University Health System / University of Hawaii, Honolulu, Hawaii
* Corresponding author. 1356 Lusitana Street, University Tower, 6th Floor, Honolulu, HI 96813.
E-mail address: timai@queens.org

Thorac Surg Clin 34 (2024) 39–49
https://doi.org/10.1016/j.thorsurg.2023.08.004
1547-4127/24/© 2023 Elsevier Inc. All rights reserved.

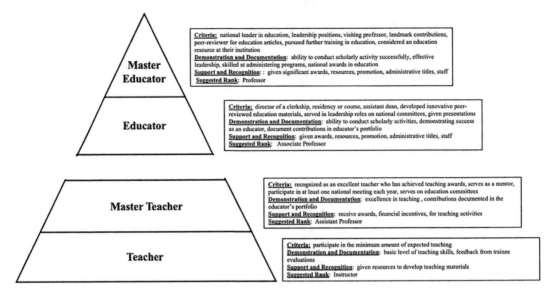

Criteria: national leader in education, leadership positions, visiting professor, landmark contributions, peer-reviewer for education articles, pursued further training in education, considered an education resource at their institution
Demonstration and Documentation: ability to conduct scholarly activity successfully, effective leadership, skilled at administering programs, national awards in education
Support and Recognition: : given significant awards, resources, promotion, administrative titles, staff
Suggested Rank: Professor

Criteria: director of a clerkship, residency or course, assistant dean, developed innovative peer-reviewed education materials, served in leadership roles on national committees, given presentations
Demonstration and Documentation: ability to conduct scholarly activities, demonstrating success as an educator, document contributions in educator's portfolio
Support and Recognition: given awards, resources, promotion, administrative titles, staff
Suggested Rank: Associate Professor

Criteria: recognized as an excellent teacher who has achieved teaching awards, serves as a mentor, participate in at least one national meeting each year, serves on education committees
Demonstration and Documentation: excellence in teaching , contributions documented in the educator's portfolio
Support and Recognition: receive awards, financial incentives, for teaching activities
Suggested Rank: Assistant Professor

Criteria: participate in the minimum amount of expected teaching
Demonstration and Documentation: basic level of teaching skills, feedback from trainee evaluations
Support and Recognition: given resources to develop teaching materials
Suggested Rank: Instructor

Fig. 1. The educators' pyramid. Classifies faculty according to their skills and achievement in education. (*Adapted from* Sachdeva et al.[3])

Today, any clinician in a health profession, who is actively engaged in both health professional and clinical activities and incorporates educational scholarship in their work, is considered a clinician-educator.[1]

DEFINING THE ROLES: TEACHER VERSUS EDUCATOR

Differentiating between the roles of teacher and educator has been ambiguous which has perpetuated a perspective where educational endeavors are not adequately recognized and rewarded. To address this challenge, the Association for Surgical Education in 1993 established a task force to further investigate the current state and identify opportunities.[3] The task force reviewed information from national sources, performed a literature review, and conducted a survey of all surgery departments in the United States and Canada. The responses reaffirmed the inadequacy of rewarding and recognizing surgeon-teachers and surgeon-educators. In addition, their investigation also confirmed that the distinction between the roles of teacher and educator was rarely made. Only 13% of respondents were able to make the distinction between "a teacher" and "an educator" in describing faulty roles.[3]

To address this result, the task force created a model, the educators' pyramid, which allows surgery faculty to be placed appropriately within a hierarchical structure that compatibly reflects their skills and levels of achievement in education. The model consists of four-tiers of hierarchy, designating the roles of teacher, master teacher, educator, and master educator. Each role contained specific criteria for placement at each level of accomplishment, methods to demonstrate and document educational contributions, and specific rewards and recognition, including suggested academic rank. The model served as a framework of criteria for appropriate recognition, reward, scholarship participation, and suggested academic rank[3] (**Fig. 1**).

SCHOLARSHIP

Scholarship is the fundamental factor that distinguishes an educator from a teacher. The most commonly adopted definition of scholarship was introduced by Earnest Boyer in 1990 as a proposal to expand the traditional definition of scholarship, which heavily focused on research (scholarship of discovery) into four types of scholarship.[4] He proposed a change in the research mission of academic institutions and by expanding the definitions of scholarship, challenged institutions to move beyond the debate between teaching and research. In addition to the scholarship of discovery, he proposed that the definition of scholarship also includes the scholarship of integration, the scholarship of application, and the scholarship of teaching and learning[4,5] (**Table 1**).

Furthermore, for to be considered scholarship, the work must meet these criteria.[6]

- The work must be made public.
- The work must be available for peer review and critique according to accepted standards.

Table 1
Types of scholarship

Types of Scholarship	Definition	Examples
Discovery	Advances knowledge	• Original published peer-reviewed research
Integration	Synthesis of information or knowledge across disciplines, topics, or time	• Interprofessional education • Patient education projects
Application	Applies disciplinary expertise or existing knowledge with results that can be shared and evaluated by peers	• Evidence-based teaching strategies • Participation in national societies • Participation on education boards and guideline panels
Teaching and Learning	Systematic investigation of teaching that is shared for review and dissemination	• Curriculum development • Preparing and delivering presentations • Develop innovative teaching modules and materials

• The work must be able to be reproduced and built on by other scholars.

Understanding scholarship and its different types is integral in the practice of an educator as it helps to define their work and achievements in education. Unlike publications of medical science research that are more readily recognized and rewarded, the work of a clinician-educator is more ambiguous. Therefore, scholarship is the work that an educator produces and how an educator can be appropriately assessed.

SKILL SETS OF AN EDUCATOR

Most faculty surgeons have a requirement to participate in some level of teaching in a variety of settings, such as in the operating room, on the wards, outpatient clinics and in the classroom. In addition, most surgeons teach based on their content expertise. However, participating in teaching and acquiring content expertise is not enough to be defined as an educator.

A surgeon using education as their academic focus requires knowledge of educational theory and formal training in how to teach effectively.[7] Being familiar with classic learning theory concepts, such as behaviorism, cognitivism, humanism, constructivism, and social learning theory help an educator understand how people learn.[8] In addition, having formal education in how these classical learning theories have evolved into frameworks of self-directed learning, transformative learning, experiential learning, and reflective practice equips

an educator to effectively apply learning theory to everyday teaching practices.

A surgeon educator must also have skills in curriculum development, instructional strategy, assessment, and educational research. These skills sets are often not taught during surgical training, and therefore, educators will often need to seek opportunities to obtain these skills outside of their clinical responsibilities.

To help surgeons develop the skills of an educator, many frameworks exist to not only define their scholarly roles but also guide one to ensure their work and initiatives are following a scholarly approach and are considered scholarship. Boyer's model of scholarship, a commonly applied and recognized framework, promotes educators to acquire skills within each category of scholarship ensuring that educators are broadly versed within their educational practices.[2] Engaging in original research that advances knowledge, clinical, or educational, fulfills the scholarship of discovery. Developing interprofessional learning opportunities, such as quality improvement projects or multidisciplinary workshops, synthesizes information and techniques across disciplines and is considered within the scholarship of integration. Practicing evidence-based teaching and implementing instructional strategies which are then followed up by evaluating and sharing the results of these initiatives accomplishes the scholarship of application. The scholarship of teaching and learning encompasses the majority of the skills and work an educator performs. It is a broad category of scholarship and can include learning through faculty development courses, curriculum development, developing innovative teaching tools, and evidence of excellence in teaching.

CLINICIAN-EDUCATOR ACADEMIC TRACKS

As more clinicians have made education the focus of their professional careers, institutions have responded by creating career tracks for academic promotion, such as the clinician-educator track. The approaches to promotion for clinician-educators can be categorized in three ways.[9]

In the first category, faculty members are primarily clinicians with some teaching responsibilities and no expectation for research. These faculty members typically are adjuncts or instructors and are rewarded if clinical expectations are met with additional service to the education mission.

Another category structures clinician-educators to hold rank in the department without tenure eligibility. This model continues to reward traditional scholarship or research, whereas the lower ranks are disproportionately filled by clinician-educators.

The third category is more equitable and creates a tenure-eligible clinician-educator track recognizing that requiring traditional scholarship is not aligned with the role of an educator. It redefines scholarship into the broader definition proposed by Boyer and rewards the appropriate duties and activities of an educator.

AN EFFECTIVE SURGICAL EDUCATOR
Knowledge Domains

Although conventional perspectives have suggested that knowledge of clinical medicine is all that is necessary to be an excellent teacher, with the ever-changing environment of health care and surgical training, knowledge of teaching skills has become equally fundamental. Surgical educators must acquire a variety of relevant knowledge domains to be an effective educator[10] (**Box 1**).

Knowledge of subject matter is perhaps the most familiar and intuitive domain that an educator pursues to acquire. The often-cited dictum of "See one, do one, teach one" tightly ties clinical expertise with the ability to teach. Many education researchers have also asserted that knowledge for teaching requires an in-depth understanding of subject matter.[11,12] In addition, a richer connection with subject matter knowledge may differentiate novice and expert teachers.[13]

Knowledge of patients is closely linked to the knowledge of subject matter. Educators must know specific facts and clinical aspects of their patients to effectively teach. This knowledge can be used to verify and assess a learner's progress and provide tips on patient care. It instills a human

Box 1
Knowledge domains of an effective surgical educator[10]
• Knowledge of subject matter
• Knowledge of patients
• Knowledge of the learners
• Knowledge of general principles of teaching and learning
• Knowledge of content-specific instruction
• Knowledge of communication

aspect in teaching and ensures quality patient care from quality instruction.[14]

Knowledge of learners enables an educator to connect learners with subject matter. This includes an understanding of the learners' prior knowledge as well as their conceptions and misconceptions of the content being taught.[10] Educators must recognize the learners' needs, motivations, and abilities.

Knowledge of principles of teaching and learning is the domain of an educator's pursuit to understand how learners learn and how instruction can be effective. Experienced educators have large repertoires of teaching strategies to be flexible in their teaching practices, enabling their ability to provide the most effective teaching environments. They recognize that learners may learn in different ways and that there is not one way to teach.

Knowledge of content-specific instruction is developed once an educator has acquired content knowledge and knowledge of teaching principles.[15] Both domains merge to transform into a new type of knowledge of content-specific instruction. This is developed through repetitive experience of teaching-specific content which becomes organized into teaching scripts. These scripts contain the goals of instruction, key teaching points, specific representations or examples, an understanding of the learners' perspectives, and procedures for overcoming learning difficulties.[16,17] Content-specific instruction is the knowledge that differentiates teachers from mere content experts.

Knowledge of communication skills exemplifies compassion, empathy, sensitivity, and intuition. Beyond being subject matter experts and skilled teachers, educators are also role models in their interactions with others. How an educator communicates in a variety of environments, differing degrees of stress, and with a variety of patients and staff is integral in not only their reception but also their effectiveness as an educator.[10]

Table 2
Domain and themes of an effective surgical educator

Domain	Theme
Attitudes intrinsic to the educator	• Promoting psychological safety • Promoting a positive learning environment • Nonthreatening • Nonjudgmental • Nonmalignant • Invested focus in the resident and their growth • Desire to teach • Patience
Behaviors intrinsic to the educator	• Good communication • Uses verbal communication to guide tasks • Nonverbal communication skills and welcoming body language • Setting goals and expectations • Regular briefing and debriefing or feedback • Deconstructing teaching into well-communicated steps • Gives autonomy • Adapting teaching to the learner
Cognitions intrinsic to the educator	• Clinical expertise • Technical expertise • Comfortable in their knowledge and skill/able to fix mistakes • Recognizes importance of teaching • Conscious effort to educate
Educator–learner relationship	• Inspirational and stimulating • Teaching residents motivates and inspires the educator • Understands their learner
Extrinsic factors	• The culture of education: good learning experiences can shape good educators

Adapted from Dickenson et al.[19]

Qualities and Traits

The qualities and traits of an effective surgical educator have been investigated from both the educator and resident perspectives. Swendiman and colleagues distributed surveys and conducted semi-structured interviews with residents and attending surgeons to identify personal qualities and teaching methods of highly effective surgical educators using a grounded theory model.[18] Personal characteristics and specific teaching approaches that facilitated successful learning included providing exceptional surgical education as a mission, strong influence from past mentors, a love for the profession, exceptional patient care, and a low-rate of self-reported burnout. Desirable teaching methods included promoting a culture of psychological safety, progressive autonomy, accountability of trainees, individualized teaching for the learner, and multimodal teaching.[18]

Another study investigating qualities and traits of an effective surgical educator focused on the resident opinion.[19] This was a qualitative and quantitative study of general surgery senior (postgraduate year 4 and 5) residents. In-depth semi-structured interviews and Likert-based survey were conducted with resident opinions undergoing thematic analysis. Five domains were developed, each containing identified themes of an effective surgical educator[19] (**Table 2**).

Intraoperative teaching effectiveness has also been investigated. Butvidas and colleagues conducted a Web-based survey asking surgeons and residents in the United States to describe their best and worst teaching experiences during training.[20] Trainee autonomy, teacher confidence, and communication were considered positive traits, whereas contemptuous, arrogant, accusatory, or uncommunicative teachers were negative behaviors. When comparing responses of the residents and attending surgeons, they found that the two groups agree on what constitutes effective and ineffective teaching in the operating room; however, they disagree on how often these behaviors occur.[20]

EDUCATION RESEARCH

Research exemplifies the scholarship of discovery and is an essential part of an educator's career and productive work. Engaging in education research differentiates an educator from a teacher. Whether it is applying education research into teaching as in the practice of evidence-based teaching or developing novel research projects as contributions to the field, education research is often an expectation for surgeons who are making surgical education their career focus. Peer-reviewed journals that focus on education include the Journal for Surgical Education,[21] Academic Medicine,[22] Medical Teacher,[23] and the Journal of Graduate Medical Education.[24] In addition, many surgical specialty journals also include a section on education topics specific for the specialty.

In many aspects, education research differs from clinical research. Most of the research in medical education focuses on reporting outcomes related to participants and has less assessment of patient care outcomes. Furthermore, the potential benefits of improved education manifest themselves over a broad set of outcomes and competencies instead of improved knowledge of specific diseases. The disease-focused structure of clinical research is more quantitative, objective, and distinct, whereas education research can be qualitative, quantitative, or have mixed methods, having more allowance for subjectivity and ambiguity.[25]

Although medical education researchers discover new knowledge and create meaningful scholarship, their work fails to be recognized within academia. Education research is often undervalued at institutions where basic science and clinical investigators are better funded, resourced, and respected.[26,27] As a result, medical education researchers face significant challenges that include lack of funding, collaborators, study subjects, and department support.

Therefore, to overcome these challenges, education researchers may need to be innovative and strategic. Gisondi and colleagues have proposed using the framework of a traditional research laboratory in conducting medical education research to overcome these challenges and increase departmental support.[28] They have developed a medical education research laboratory start-up guide that includes steps of identifying a leader or leaders, set a vision and a mission, choose organizational structure, identify resource and infrastructure needs, and identify funding mechanisms. In addition, to obtain funding for medical education research, researchers may need to be creative, flexible, and adaptive in presenting their ideas in ways that are appealing and relevant to the goals of funders.[29]

ACQUIRING THE SKILLS, QUALIFICATIONS, AND CREDENTIALS

Despite the fundamental role and responsibilities of preparing graduates for unsupervised practice, surgical educators often receive little formal education to help prepare them for these complex roles. The knowledge and skills required are not covered in the current standard surgical training paradigm. In addition, accreditation bodies are also increasingly requiring their residency leaders to have "requisite specialty expertise and documented educational and administrative experience."[30,31] Therefore, to meet these challenges, it is necessary for surgical educators to often pursue educational opportunities, outside of their clinical practices, to develop additional competencies in education.[31,32]

American College of Surgeons: Surgeons as Educators

The Surgeons as Educators course is a week-long intensive, full-time course organized annually by the American College of Surgeons Division of Education and has been offered for 27 years. Participants are provided knowledge and skills to enhance their abilities as teachers, leaders, and administrators of surgical education programs. The course equips participants with strategies and tools to develop effective learning environments for medical students, surgical residents, surgical fellows, and colleagues. It is designed for full-time faculty members who are interested in acquiring skills in curriculum development, teaching, performance and program evaluation, and program administration.

Association for Surgical Education: Surgical Education Research Fellowship

Surgical Education Research Fellowship (SERF) was founded in 1980 and is a 1-year fellowship for faculty interested in pursuing educational research. The fellowship is designed to equip investigators with the skills and knowledge needed to plan, implement, and report research studies in surgical education. Each SERF fellow is matched with an advisor and culminates with a completed project ready for presentation at the Association for Surgical Education annual meeting and submission to a peer-reviewed journal.

American College of Surgeons: Residents as Teachers and Leaders

Surgical residency is tailored for residents to master clinical and basic science knowledge as well as operative skills. However, residents are also expected to master several critical nonclinical skills, such as leading teams and teaching. Because very few residency programs offer opportunities for residents to become proficient in these areas, the American College of Surgeons Division of Education offers a 3-day course to address these needs. The content of the course focuses on skills for residents' lifelong roles as teachers, leaders, and practicing surgeons.

Surgical Education and Simulation Research Fellowship at Accredited Education Institutes-Accredited Fellowship Programs

The Fellowship Program of the Consortium of ACS-Accredited Education Institutes (AEI) was established to improve the quality of surgical care by developing future leaders and scholars in the area of surgical education, simulation, and training. A handful of ACS AEI programs within the country offer these accredited fellowships and each has their own selection criteria, curriculum, and requirements for completion. Common curricular content focuses on simulation-based education and the application of health care simulation into the participant's future career. In addition, this is one of the few fellowship opportunities that welcome resident applicants.

American College of Surgeons: Certificate in Applied Surgical Education Leadership

The Certificate in Applied Surgical Education Leadership offered by the American College of Surgeons Division of Education is an opportunity for participants to receive additional formal training to further develop specific skills necessary to be a leader in surgical education. This is an extending learning course as applicants are required to have completed the ACS Surgeons as Educators course or equivalent which may include the SERF Program, advanced medical education certificate, or advanced degree program. The goals of the program are to prepare participants for leadership roles in surgical education, impact quality and patient safety through surgical education, and improve surgical education by promoting innovation and change. By the end of the year-long program, applicants are required to complete a surgical education leadership project at their home institution.

Association of Surgical Education: Surgical Education and Leadership Fellowship

Surgical Education and Leadership Fellowship is a 1-year fellowship designed for members of the Association of Surgical Education to improve their teaching, education design, and leadership skills in surgical education. Participants are assigned an experienced advisor who provides coaching and tools necessary to enhance abilities as teachers and leaders in surgical education.

Advanced Degrees

With increasing need for educators and educational leaders, several advanced degree and graduate programs in health care professions education are now offered. The two most common degrees are the Masters in Education for Healthcare Professions and the Masters in Healthcare Professions Education (MHPE). Thirty years ago, there were few MHPE programs; in 2013, there were 121 programs; and in 2018, there were 150 programs worldwide.[31] Although the content of each program may vary, most master's degree programs are competency-based educational experiences focusing on adult learning theory, research, and the practice and application of education as it applies to health professions environments. The core content is often categorized into the five domains of educational activity: (1) teaching and learning, (2) curriculum development, (3) program evaluation, (4) educational research methods, and (5) leadership and management.[31] MHPE programs are offered in two formats, in-person courses on campus or the online format, and can be often completed in 2 to 4 years. Course schedules and work are designed to allow students to complete the degree while keeping their full-time employment positions.

The primary difference between a certificate program and a master's degree is the common MHPE graduation requirement of conducting original research as a capstone project, which is submitted for publication in a peer-reviewed journal,[31] whereas certificate programs typically involve only coursework and participation as a practicum experience.

BUILDING A NATIONAL REPUTATION AS AN EDUCATOR

Organizations that are devoted specifically to surgical education are the Association for Surgical Education, the Association of Program Directors in Surgery, and the American College of Surgeons Division of Education. In addition, the Thoracic Surgery Directors Association (TSDA) serves as an organization specifically for cardiothoracic surgical education and the Association of American Medical Colleges (AAMC) has a broader focus, including opportunities for undergraduate, graduate, and continuing medical education. These organizations have annual meetings that offer workshops, career development programs, opportunities to learn about advances in surgical education, networking opportunities, and resources for identifying mentors.

Furthermore, many of these organizations also allow surgical educators to improve their visibility at a national level. They often will provide networking opportunities and are an excellent resource for identifying mentors within education. In addition, there are opportunities to participate in various committees and serve in leadership positions. Overall, membership in organizations with an education mission allows an educator to find communities of practice for peer support, mentorship, sponsorship, resources, and best practices.[32]

In 2017, the American College of Surgeons launched the Academy of Master Surgeon Educators and inducted its first group of members in 2018. Members of the Academy are selected through a rigorous peer-review process, recognizing dedication, a commitment to excellence, and advancement of the science and practice of surgical education. The aim of the Academy is to assemble a cadre of renowned master surgeon educators who will work closely and engage in activities with the American College of Surgeons Division of Education.

DOCUMENTING AN EDUCATOR'S WORK
Making Education Activity Count

Many educational activities are not captured by the traditional curriculum vitae, and therefore, educators' contributions to their institutions may not be appropriately recognized. In 2006, a Consensus Conference on Educational Scholarship was convened by the AAMC Group on Education Affairs to outline and develop documentation standards for use by educators and academic promotion committees.[33] The investigators emphasized that educational excellence requires documentation of the quantity and quality of education activities. They recommended that education activity documentation include.[33]

- A brief description of the activity and the educator's role
- Evidence of quantity for each activity which includes who is being taught, how many learners, what is being taught, when, where and how often is the activity and how much time was devoted to the activity.
- Evidence of quality describing the effectiveness and outcomes of the activity. Evidence may include evaluations, peer review ratings, learner comments, invitations to teach outside one's own department and/or institution, impact on learner performance demonstrated

by pre-post improvement in test scores, and sustainability of the curriculum.
- Evidence of engagement with the education community describing how the educator's work is informed by what is known in the existing literature, best practices, and resources, how the work draws on resources such as grant funding, and how the work is made visible and disseminated.

Educational Portfolio

In addition to documenting specific education activities, a teaching or education portfolio is used to display and organize all the work an educator produces. A common framework for developing an education portfolio consists of the following components.[34]

- Teaching philosophy or reflective statement
- Introductory statement describing teaching responsibilities, roles, and positions
- Material representative of teaching practices
- Teaching awards and recognition
- Professional development efforts
- Appendix: additional evaluative material

The teaching philosophy is a 1-page reflective statement of the educator's perspective on teaching and how they will apply that perspective into their teaching practices. It describes the educator's beliefs about teaching and learning. The teaching philosophy should include the educator's core ideas about being an effective teacher and explain why they have chosen these ideals. The teaching philosophy is an opportunity for the educator to share their past experiences in teaching or being taught and how they have developed their teaching beliefs from these experiences.

The introductory statement is a brief narrative defining the educator's roles. It should also include teaching responsibilities, percentage of effort devoted to teaching and courses taught. The introductory statement offers details describing who are the learners the educator teaches (faculty, residents, fellows, medical students), where they are teaching (inpatient floors, clinics, operating room, simulation center), and what are they teaching (patient care skills, technical skills, interpersonal communication skills). In addition, the scholarly focus of the educator or education "specialty" can also be described, such as curriculum development, technology, simulation, accreditation, assessment, diversity/inclusion, and quality improvement.

The material representative of teaching practices section comprises the majority of the portfolio. It is meant to be descriptive and detailed so the work of the educator can be fully appreciated and assessed. This is where a variety of teaching activities can be described and included. Examples of teaching activities include formal curricula developed by the educator, creation of teaching material, assessment and survey validation, course development, education research projects and publications, and evidence of mentorship. The framework proposed by the Consensus Conference on Educational Scholarship, as described prior, can be used to thoroughly document educational activities.[33]

One component of the teaching awards and recognition section includes awards given for excellence in teaching. In addition, this section also includes invited lectureships and visiting professorships on education topics. Educational administration and leadership endeavors, including service on advisory and examination boards, are also included. Award funding or scholarship awards are listed with a description of not only the award but also the award process. Appointment to leadership positions within institutional, regional, and national societies and committees focusing on education can be stated in this section as well as membership in societies recognizing achievements in education such as the American College of Surgeons Academy of Master Surgeon Educators.

Professional development efforts include the endeavors that an educator has engaged to further improve their teaching practices and learn about advances in education and collaborations fostering innovation in education. Examples include attendance in faculty development workshops, participating in continuing medical education courses, completing education fellowships, acquiring certifications in specific areas of education, and coursework for achieving advanced degrees in education.

The appendix section serves as a section which includes other work within education that may not "fit" within the other sections but may be important for the educator to document, such as annual teaching evaluations.

EVALUATING THE WORK OF AN EDUCATOR

For clinician-educators, making their education activities visible and valued is a challenge in institutions that are dependent on research grants and clinical revenue. However, educators must be supported and rewarded to sustain the educational mission of academic institutions. Therefore, as institutional leaders increasingly recognize education in academic advancement, determining standards in the evaluation of educator activities must be established.

To promote a fair process in the evaluation of educators, in 2010, the Association of American Medical Colleges (AAMC) Task Force on Educator Evaluation was formed to establish consensus guidelines for use by those responsible for evaluating educational contributions of faculty.[35] The purpose of the guidelines was to serve as an objective method for rigorous evaluation of educators that can be used by institutions to support faculty who have chosen to focus their careers in education. By using an evidence-based framework, the Task Force created the Toolbox for Evaluating Educators, which contains criteria to evaluate faculty in each of the five domains of educator activity. Prior work by Simpson and colleagues established these domains as the most common sets of educational activity documented in teaching portfolios of faculty in 16 US academic institutions.[33] The five domains include teaching, curriculum development, advising and mentoring, education leadership and administration, and learner assessment.[36] The Task Force then applied Glassick's criteria for the assessment of scholarship and recommended that each educational incorporate clear goals, adequate preparation, appropriate methods, significant results, effective presentation, and reflective critique.[5,36]

ADVANCEMENT AND PROMOTION

Academic advancement has been slower for clinician-educators than for faculty involved in traditional research.[37] The role that educational endeavors play in the academic advancement of faculty is often poorly defined. A cross-sectional survey was distributed to the membership of the Association for Surgical Education to identify factors associated with promotion for faculty pursuing education scholarship as their academic focus.[37] Advanced academic rank was associated with male gender, advanced age, publication of education topics, funding for research in education, recipient of teaching awards, and status as an officer in an education association.

In another investigation, senior academic surgeons who are members of the Society of University Surgeons and the Society of Surgical Chairs were surveyed to develop an expert consensus on criteria for academic promotion.[38]

The three categories of activity that were most highly rated for promotion to associate professor were (1) scholarship, (2) teaching, and (3) administration. The three most highly ranked criteria for promotion to the associate level were:

1. Active participation in conferences/departmental educational activities

2. Education portfolio demonstrates commitment to activities as an educator.
3. Clinical teaching excellence at home institution

The median number of publications was 10 for promotion to associate professor.

For promotion to professor, the most highly rated categories of activity were (1) scholarship, (2) administration, and (3) teaching and mentorship. The three most highly ranked criteria for promotion to professor were.

1. Mentorship of junior surgical educators
2. Active participation in conferences/departmental educational activities
3. Record of teaching excellence

The median number of publications was 22.5 for promotion to professor.

SUMMARY

The surgical educator academic track is different from a surgical scientist track in terms of skills, work performed, documentation, and promotion requirements. A cardiothoracic surgery educator not only has the passion to teach but must also go beyond the "I love to teach" perspective, having a dedicated effort and active practice of scholarship.

CLINICS CARE POINTS

- The roles of teacher and educator are different
- An educator actively practices scholarship
- For work to be defined as scholarship, it must be made public, available for peer review and critique, and reproducible and built on by other scholars

DISCLOSURE

A.W. Wong and T.A. Imai: no disclosure.

REFERENCES

1. Greenberg L. The evolution of the clinician-educator in the United States and Canada: personal reflections over the last 45 years. Acad Med 2018; 93(12):1764–6.
2. Branch WT, Kroenke K, Levinson W. The clinician-educator- present and future roles. J Gen Intern Med 1997;12(suppl 2):S1–4.
3. Sachdeva AK, Cohen R, Dayton MT, et al. A new model for recognizing and rewarding the educational accomplishments of surgery faculty. Acad Med 1999;74(12):1278–87.
4. Boyer EL. Scholarship reconsidered: priorities of the professoriate. Princeton, NJ: The Carnegie Foundation for the Advancement of Teaching; 1990.
5. Glassick CE. Boyer's expanded definitions of scholarship, the standards for assessing scholarship, and the elusiveness of the scholarship of teaching. Acad Med 2000;75(9):877–80.
6. Shulman L. The scholarship of teaching. Change 1999;31(5):11.
7. Khan N, Khan MS, Dasgupta P, et al. The surgeon as educator: fundamentals of faculty training in surgical specialties. BJU Int 2012;111:171–8.
8. Wilkerson L, Irby DM. Strategies for improving teaching practices: a comprehensive approach to faculty development. Acad Med 1998;73(4):387–96.
9. Fleming VM, Schindler N, Martin GJ, et al. Separate and equitable promotion tracks for clinician-educators. JAMA 2005;294(9):1101–4.
10. Irby DM. What clinical teachers in medicine need to know. Acad Med 1994;69(5):333–42.
11. Brophy J. Teachers' knowledge of subject matter as it relates to their teaching practice. Greenwich (CT): JAI Press; 1991.
12. Grossman PL, Wilson SM, Shulman LS. Teachers of substance: subject matter knowledge for teaching. In: Reynolds MC, editor. Knowledge Base for the Beginning teacher. New York: Pergamon Press; 1989. p. 245–64.
13. Leinhardt G. Math lessons: a contrast of novice and expert competence. J Res Math Educ 1989;20:52–75.
14. Matter WD, Weinholtz D, Friedman CP. The attending physician as teacher. N Engl J Med 1983;308:1129–32.
15. Shulman L. Those who understand: knowledge growth in teaching. Educ Res 1986;15:4–14.
16. Putnam RT. Structuring and adjusting content for students: a study of live and simulated tutoring of addition. Am Educ Res J 1987;24:13–48.
17. Gudmundsdottir S. Pedagogicla models of subject matter. In: Teachers' knowledge of subject matter as it relates to their teaching practice. Greenwich (CT): JAI Press; 1991.
18. Swendiman RA, Hoffman DI, Bruce AN, et al. Qualities and methods of highly effective surgical educators: A grounded theory model. J Surg Educ 2011; 201:385–9.
19. Dickenson KJ, Bass BL, Pei KY. What embodies an effective surgical educator? A grounded theory analysis of resident opinion. Surgery 2020;168:730–6.
20. Butvidas LD, Anderson CI, Balough D, et al. Disparities between resident and attending surgeon perceptions of intraoperative teaching. Am J Surg 2011;201:385–9.

21. Journal of Surgical Education. Available at: http://www.elsevier.com/wps/find/journaldescription.cws_home/710600/authorinstructions. Accessed: May 31, 2023.
22. Academic Medicine. Available at: http://journals.lww.com/academicmedicine/pages/default.aspx. Accessed: May 31, 2023.
23. Medical Teacher. Available at: http://www.medicalteacher.org. Accessed May 31, 2023.
24. Journal of Graduate Medical Education. Available at: https://meridian.allenpress.com/jgme. Accessed May 31, 2023.
25. Ringsted C, Hodges B, Scherpbier A. The research compass': an introduction to research in medical education: AMEE Guide No. 56. Med Teach 2011; 33(9):695–709.
26. Hu WC, Thistlethwaite JE, Weller J, et al. It was serendipity: a qualitative study of academic careers in medical education. Med Educ 2015;49:1124–36.
27. Irby DM, O'Sullivan PS. Developing and rewarding teachers as educators and scholars: remarkable progress and daunting challenges. Med Educ 2018;52:58–67.
28. Gisondi MA, Michael S, Li-Sauerwine S, et al. The purpose, design and promise of medical education research labs. Acad Med 2022;97(9):1281–8.
29. Gruppen LD, Durning SJ. Needles and Haystacks: Finding funding for medical education research. Acad Med 2016;91(4):480–4.
30. Accreditation Council for Graduate Medical Education. ACGME Common Program Requirements. Available at: https://www.acgme.org/Portals/0/PFAssets/ProgramRequirements/CPRs_2017-07-01.pdf. Accessed May 31, 2023.
31. Artino AR, Cervero RM, DeZee KJ, et al. Graduate programs in health professions education: preparing academic leaders for future challenges. J Grad Med Educ 2018;10(2):119–22.
32. Sanfey H, Boehler M, DaRosa D, et al. Career development resource: educational leadership in a department of surgery: vice chairs for education. Am J Surg 2012;204:121–5.
33. Simpson D, Fincher RM, Hafler JP, et al. Advancing educators and education by defining the components and evidence associated with educational scholarship. Med Educ 2007;41:1002–9.
34. Sanfey H, Gantt NL. Career development resource: academic career in surgical education. Am J Surg 2012;204:126–9.
35. Gusic ME, Baldwin CD, Chandran L, et al. Evaluating educators using a novel toolbox: applying rigorous criteria flexibly across institutions. Acad Med 2014;89(7):1006–11.
36. Simpson D, Hafler J, Brown D, et al. Documentation systems for educators seeking academic promotion in US medical schools. Acad Med 2004;79:783–90.
37. Klingensmith ME, Anderson KD. Educational scholarship as a route to academic promotion: a depiction of surgical education scholars. Am J Surg 2006;191:533–7.
38. Cochran A, Neumayer LA, Mellinger JD, et al. Career advancement for surgeon-educators: findings from a modified Delphi process. J Surg Educ 2021;79(1):173–8.

Navigating Promotion in Thoracic Surgery

Marko T. Boskovski, MD, MHS, MPH, Elaine E. Tseng, MD*

KEYWORDS

- Academic promotion • Clinical excellence • Funding • Education • Teaching • Digital scholarship
- Community service • Diversity, equity, and inclusion

KEY POINTS

- The promotion process at academic institutions is clearly defined, and a thorough understanding of the promotion process is the key to successful advancement in academia.
- Promotion criteria vary based on academic tracks.
- Regardless of track, typically assistant professors garner regional recognition, associate professors achieve national recognition and full professors have international acclaim.
- Promotion criteria can include but are not limited to clinical excellence, research/investigation, funding, education/teaching, service to the community, academic center, professional organizations and the lay public, health policy, diversity, equity, and inclusion, ethics, quality and safety, and health care delivery.
- Promotion packets, which should be updated regularly, include components such as CVs, narrative statements, letters of support, and teaching portfolios.

INTRODUCTION

The lifespan of academic physicians can be rich and diverse, yet to many young physicians starting out, it can also appear shrouded in mystery. How does one move successfully through the promotion process while maintaining self-efficacy and work satisfaction? The key lies in an early and thorough understanding of the promotion process, leading to meaningful, goal-driven professional pursuits.

Overview of the Promotion Process

The journey begins with an initial, postgraduate faculty appointment within one's home department or division. Depending on the institution, this typically begins at the rank of instructor or assistant professor.

At most academic medical centers, there exist multiple tracks for promotion, each with its own specific guidelines and requirements of accomplishments.[1] An inclusive but not exhaustive list of such tracks includes clinical, investigative, educational, administrative, or combination tracks with more differentiated areas of concentrations. It is therefore essential to gain a clear understanding of what counts as *scholarship* for each track and how such various academic contributions are valued.[2] For example, National Institutes of Health (NIH) funding will likely be heavily weighted when considering promotion for investigative tracks, whereas curricula development may count for educational tracks and the development of new clinical protocols important for clinical tracks.[3] It is also helpful to know institution-specific submission deadlines for planning purposes, such as obtaining references and teaching evaluations in a timely manner. Some institutions may have length of service requirements, with the possibility of "early" promotion for exceptional candidates. Institutions should have clear and detailed guidelines of their promotion process readily available, either in print, online, or by request from the Office of Academic Affairs or Office of Faculty Affairs.[4,5]

Division of Adult Cardiothoracic Surgery, Department of Surgery, University of California San Francisco and San Francisco VA Medical Center, 500 Parnassus Avenue, MUW 405, Box 0118, San Francisco, CA 94143, USA
* Corresponding author.
E-mail address: elaine.tseng@ucsf.edu

Thorac Surg Clin 34 (2024) 51–56
https://doi.org/10.1016/j.thorsurg.2023.08.005
1547-4127/24/Published by Elsevier Inc.

However, less than one-quarter of US medical schools had above average documentation for promotion and tenure.[2]

Criteria for Advancement

There are many ways in which the promotions committee assesses readiness of a faculty candidate for promotion. Metrics will vary and become more rigorous with ascending rank. The following discussions paint broad strokes of typical requirements, but specifics will vary depending on the institution.

Clinical Excellence

Clinical competence is necessary but not sufficient for rise through the academic ranks. Developing a particular clinical niche within cardiothoracic surgery is of critical importance, as it allows faculty members to focus their efforts and energy on a particular area of clinical expertise or innovation, such that they may garner regional, national, or international recognition. The development of such a niche may go hand in hand with the development of clinical programs and leadership roles. Furthermore, expertise in a niche is likely to lead to invitations for talks or other modes of scholarship dissemination, clinical leadership roles, and awards for clinical contributions. Irrespective of whether one's track is clinical, research, or teaching/mentoring, the area of clinical expertise ideally corresponds to one's clinical or research publications in that same field to demonstrate a focused area of concentration.

Research/Investigation

This category pertains to research in a traditional sense, acknowledging that research and innovation can and occurs in all other categories discussed later in this review.

Mural and extramural funding plays a central role in the promotion process of faculty in research/investigation tracks. The attainment of a commensurate level of funding may be required for academic promotion. Furthermore, the funding itself provides necessary resources for scholarly activity that yields peer-reviewed publications, which are highly valued in the promotion process.

Instructor and assistant professor-level research faculty in thoracic surgery typically start off with early-career foundation grants from societies such as the Thoracic Surgery Foundation (TSF), American Association for Thoracic Surgery (AATS), American Heart Association (AHA), and others.[6–9] A significant portion of cardiothoracic surgeons is not eligible for career development awards (CDAs), such as AHA or veterans affairs (VA) CDA, or NIH K awards, as they require a 75% effort that is difficult to obtain in most divisions.[10,11] Thus, early to mid-career faculty who have successfully obtained funding from foundation grants often face a "mid-career" funding drought in their quest for R01 level funding, when the foundation grants expire. If start-up funds were made available to young faculty on recruitment, one strategy may be to first seek and use foundation grants, then use start-up funds as a bridge until R01 or equivalent (VA merit) funding can be obtained.

Associate and full professor-level research faculty are typically expected to have independent research laboratories with R01 or equivalent funding. Foundations in the thoracic surgery field (TSF and AATS) have recognized the difficulties of this transition to R01 funding. As such, they have extended their early investigator award applications up to 7 years of completion of residency unlike the traditional expectation of within 4 years of faculty appointment. In addition, mid-career awards have been offered in selected settings to support diversity, equity, and inclusion (DEI). Building and growing a basic science laboratory while maintaining an active clinical practice can be a challenging endeavor. Partnership with PhD professors is a well-recognized approach in divisions of cardiothoracic surgery to remain at the forefront of academic research. Nonetheless, other research avenues include obtaining Masters in public health with specialized training in biostatistics for clinical investigation, followed by participation in multicenter randomized clinical trials either through the NIH/VA or industry-sponsored trials. Although junior faculty often begin as coinvestigators, they can transition into leadership roles as site-principal investigators (PIs) for their institutions. Further development in this track allows mid-career faculty to create, develop, and lead randomized multicenter clinical trials as PIs through either the NIH Cardiothoracic Surgery Network or the VA Collaborative Studies Program. Industry sponsored clinical trials are more often developed by industry to evaluate pharmaceuticals or devices with surgeon leadership in clinical endpoints and conduct of the trials. As such, conflicts of interest and codes of ethics are particularly pertinent in such relationships with industry.[12] Both basic science and clinical research allow demonstration of productivity in the medical literature.

Contributions to the medical literature can take many forms, the most common being peer-reviewed publications. The number of publications is important, as are the type of authorship and the impact factor of the publication. The number of first or last author publications has been shown to be directly correlated with rank.[13] Some institutions use the "h-index" as a "personal impact factor," which measures both the productivity and the citation impact of one's cumulative publications.[13,14] Other scholarly contributions include books, chapters, lectures, and workshops.

Education/Teaching

Substantive contributions to education are a main tenet of the promotion process given its centrality to the academic mission. This is a wide-reaching category of contribution that includes both clinical and didactic teaching, with a wide target audience that can include medical students, health professions students, residents, fellows and peers, whereas research teaching can include college and graduate MS and PhD students as well as postdoctoral fellows and junior research faculty.

Education can also take the form of contributions to curricula, publications in clinical teaching or medical education, and service on education-related committees.

Many institutions require a teaching portfolio for promotion. These portfolios typically include a summation of teaching evaluations, and if applicable, curricular developments, educational scholarship, mentoring, evidence of regional/national/international recognition and educational leadership.[1,15] Leadership roles within the teaching and mentoring arena can include Residency Director positions at the institution, faculty participation nationally in the Thoracic Surgery Directors Association, where as early as residency, resident leaders can participate in the Thoracic Surgery Resident Association. Similarly other leadership roles can include service to the American Board of Thoracic Surgery as an Oral Board Examiner.

Digital Scholarship

Digital scholarship is a relatively new arena of scholarly contribution that has been increasingly used since the COVID-19 pandemic, during which time many physicians turned to social media and digital platforms to disseminate and communicate health information and scholarly work. This growing trend is likely to be increasingly reflected in promotion considerations, as institutions develop more objective metrics and evaluation processes for what merits inclusion as scholarship.[16,17]

Service to the Community, Academic Center, Professional Organizations, and the Lay Public

These categories may overlap with some already mentioned, including service on organizations within the university, including administrative or leadership positions within the academic center. Faculty may serve the university and department though committees such as medical school admissions, institutional review boards, intramural grants, clinical competence, residency review, faculty recruitment search committees, and academic senate committees among others. Senior faculty are requested on promotions committees as well as leadership roles within the academic senate. Extramurally, service to professional organizations such as the AHA, Society of Thoracic Surgeons, TSF, AATS, NIH, and so forth through societal committees can result in leadership opportunities within those organizations. Activities can include participating in the leadership committees, organizing annual scientific meetings, grading abstracts, organizing sessions, and moderating at scientific meetings, participating and/or leading grant review committees, fund raising, and outreach. Thoracic surgery journals, such as Annals of Thoracic Surgery, and Journal of Thoracic and Cardiovascular Surgery among others also provide ample opportunities for service including reviewing publications, serving on editorial boards, and providing thoughtful invited commentaries. Last, volunteer activities within the patient community and development of educational materials for the lay public also are important services to the broader patient population.

Additional Categories

Faculty may also have a substantial body of work in other realms, such as health policy, DEI, ethics, quality and safety, and health care delivery. A comprehensive list would not be possible given the exhaustive possibilities. Contributions in these realms are important and not considered diminutive in comparison to more traditional categories of promotion but merely reflect a smaller proportion of candidates advancing through excellence in these categories. However, it is important to understand the guidelines at each specific institution to understand how such accomplishments are weighed, and whether or not they are considered a substitute for other metrics.

Letters of Support

Requirements will vary based on proposed rank, but letters of reference will be required from both internal and external evaluators. Internal evaluators may also be requested from faculty in other departments. This is meant to compare one's productivity against others holding similar appointments in the cardiothoracic (CT) surgery. Developing mentors from other departments can helpful with obtaining a more balanced perspective regarding the promotion process and are important to have outside the traditional senior surgical mentors. These evaluators should be at or above the rank of one's proposed promotion. Think early and keep internal lists of individuals who are leaders in CT surgery at other institutions who are knowledgeable about your work and contributions.

Curriculum Vitae and Narrative Statement

Think of the curriculum vitae as the autobiography of one's academic career: this should be tended to frequently and with care and precision. Using institution-specific formatting will make the process easier, as they tend to outline critical portions needed by your institution. Most institutions also require a narrative statement, harkening back to the days of medical school and residency applications. Update this annually with any shifts in career aspirations and accomplishments to maintain coherence.

Up the Ladder: Assistant to Associate to Professor

Although specific requirements will vary by institution, the promotion process up the ranks can be thought of in broad strokes as increasing demands on scholarship, teaching, and service and increasing renown for one's clinical or scholastic contributions.

Generally, in order to be promoted to the rank of assistant professor, one must show promise of achieving renown in one's field. Assistant professors typically garner regional recognition, with the potential to develop into an excellent educator, clinician, and/or researcher. Publications may be mostly first author, with emerging last author status. The allocation of weight to each category will vary, and it is important to work closely with mentors to ensure that one is appropriately allocating time to various activities.

In order to rise to the rank of associate professor, one must achieve national recognition for one's creative, scholarly or research activities. This may mean independent extramural research funding, status as PI, and more senior author publications. Clinically, one may have developed innovative methods of disease management or new surgical techniques, or spearheaded a center of excellence in a particular surgical procedure. Typically, at the associate level, one is expected to make significant contributions of service, either through sitting on department or university committees or national professional organizations.

Appointment to professor requires further professional development and excellence in clinical care and teaching. At this level, one is expected to have national and international renown related to scholarly activities.

Diversity, Equity, and Inclusion in the Promotion Process

Although academic intuitions are heavily invested in faculty promotion and advancement, this process is not without challenges.

Underrepresented in medicine (URiM) physicians are less likely to get the promoted and have a higher probability of attrition from academic faculty positions.[18] Furthermore, URiM faculty report more debt and are more likely to need to supplement their income, which may take time away from academic pursuits and lead to attrition from academia altogether.[19]

Additional challenges include the lack of clarity about the promotion process, perceiving promotion criteria as too stringent and perceived disparities and inequities among advancement tracks. Although many institutions are also becoming more aware of these factors contributing to burnout and attrition among faculty, many of these concerns remain problematic, especially among early career, non-white and female faculty.[20]

Although women constitute over one-half of medical school graduates, there is significant underrepresentation of women in surgery.[21] However, women are significantly less likely to be interested in thoracic surgery, and only 7% of thoracic surgeons were women in 2017—the lowest compared with all other surgical subspecialties.[22–24] Furthermore, there are even fewer women in higher academic ranks and leadership positions.[25] Thus, female faculty are less likely to be full professors and division chiefs compared with men. Female cardiothoracic surgeons had fewer publications than men, and this was most pronounced at the assistant professor level. However, this did not translate to lower NIH funding, as men and women had similar rates of past and present grant funding.[26–29]

Although women have fewer publications than men, especially at lower academic ranks, female faculty often perform better than their male counterparts at senior faculty positions, suggesting that women have potential for career peaks later in their careers. Furthermore, in surgery publications authored by women have greater impact, and better NIH-funded departments have a higher fraction of female full professors.[26,30,31]

SUMMARY

Although the academic promotion process may seem complicated at the outset, once it is broken down into granular steps, it should appear clearer and less daunting. Young faculty can take the lead on their careers by being visible and proactive within their departments and institutions. Connecting with mentors and departmental leadership early can help the physician better understand what is defined as "scholarship" and "excellence," as every institution has different nuanced philosophies and valued traditions. One should establish frequent check-ins with these mentors and regularly update *curriculum vitae* with accomplishments. When the definition of excellence is clear, and the effort toward achieving that excellence is well-directed, the stress of academic promotion may be lessened and work satisfaction increased.

FUNDING

Elaine Tseng was funded by the Marfan Foundation and Veterans Affairs Merit Award I01CX002365-01A1.

DISCLOSURE

The authors have nothing to disclose.

REFERENCES

1. Fleming VM, Schindler N, Martin GJ, et al. Separate and Equitable Promotion Tracks for Clinician-Educators. JAMA 2005;294(9):1101.
2. Hoffman LA, Lufler RS, Brown KM, et al. A review of U.S. Medical schools' promotion standards for educational excellence. Teach Learn Med 2020; 32(2):184–93.
3. Guadalupe FM, Knox KS. Principles of Academic Life: Appointment, Promotion, and Tenure. Available at: https://www.aamc.org/professional-development/affinity-groups/gfa/principles-academic-life-appointment-promotion-and-tenure. Accessed April 29, 2023.
4. A Faculty Handbook for Success: Advancement and Promotion at UCSF. Available at: https://senate.ucsf.edu/sites/default/files/2016-12/FacultyHandbook-UCSF.pdf. Accessed April 29, 2023.
5. Harvard Medical School Office for Faculty Affairs Promotion Profile Library. Available at: https://fa.hms.harvard.edu/promotion-profile-library. Accessed April 29, 2023.
6. Aranda-Michel E, Luketich JD, Rao R, et al. The effect of receiving an award from the American Association for Thoracic Surgery Foundation. JTCVS Open 2022;10:282–9.
7. The Thoracic Surgery Foundation Awards. Available at: https://thoracicsurgeryfoundation.org/awards/. Accessed April 29, 2023.
8. American Association of Thoracic Surgery Foundation Programs. Available at: https://www.aats.org/foundation. Accessed April 29, 2023.
9. American Heart Association Career Development Award. Available at: https://professional.heart.org/en/research-programs/aha-funding-opportunities/career-development-award. Accessed April 29, 2023.
10. National Institutes of Health Research Career Development Awards. Available at: https://researchtraining.nih.gov/programs/career-development. Accessed April 29, 2023.
11. U.S. Department of Veterans Affairs Office of Research & Development Career Development Program. Available at: https://www.research.va.gov/funding/cdp.cfm. Accessed April 29, 2023.
12. Mack MJ, Sade RM, American Association for Thoracic Surgery Ethics Committee, et al. Relations Between Cardiothoracic Surgeons and Industry. Ann Thorac Surg 2009;87(5):1334–6.
13. Cheng TW, Farber A, Rajani RR, et al. National criteria for academic appointment in vascular surgery. J Vasc Surg 2019;69(5):1559–65.
14. Ashfaq A, Kalagara R, Wasif N. H-index and academic rank in general surgery and surgical specialties in the United States. J Surg Res 2018;229:108–13.
15. Schwarz F, Baumann P, Manthey J, et al. The effect of aortic valve replacement on survival. Circulation 1982;66(5):1105–10.
16. Cabrera D, Roy D, Chisolm MS. Social Media Scholarship and Alternative Metrics for Academic Promotion and Tenure. J Am Coll Radiol 2018;15(1):135–41.
17. Johng SY, Mishori R, Korostyshevskiy VR. Social media, digital scholarship, and academic promotion in us medical schools. Fam Med 2021;53(3):215–9.
18. Liu CQ, Alexander H. The changing demographics of full-time U.S. Medical School Faculty; 2011. Available at: https://www.aamc.org/media/5931/download. Accessed April 30, 2023.
19. Jeffe DB, Yan Y, Andriole DA. Competing Risks Analysis of Promotion and Attrition in Academic Medicine: A National Study of U.S. Medical School Graduates. Acad Med 2019;94(2):227–36.
20. Tung J, Nahid M, Rajan M, et al. The impact of a faculty development program, the Leadership in Academic Medicine Program (LAMP), on self-efficacy, academic promotion and institutional retention. BMC Med Educ 2021;21(1). https://doi.org/10.1186/s12909-021-02899-y.
21. Heiser S. The Majority of U.S. Medical Students Are Women, New Data Show. Available at: https://www.aamc.org/news-insights/press-releases/majority-us-medical-students-are-women-new-data-show. Accessed April 30, 2023.
22. Zhuge Y, Kaufman J, Simeone DM, et al. Is there still a glass ceiling for women in academic surgery? Ann Surg 2011;253(4):637–43.
23. Aziz HA, Ducoin C, Welsh DJ, et al. 2018 American College of Surgeons Governors Survey: Gender inequality and harassment remain a challenge in

surgery. Available at: https://bulletin.facs.org/2019/09/2018-acs-governors-survey-gender-inequality-and-harassment-remain-a-challenge-in-surgery/#. Accessed April 30, 2023.

24. Miller VM, Padilla LA, Swicord WB, et al. Gender Differences in Cardiothoracic Surgery Interest Among General Surgery Applicants. Ann Thorac Surg 2021;112(3):961–7.

25. Abelson JS, Chartrand G, Moo TA, et al. The climb to break the glass ceiling in surgery: trends in women progressing from medical school to surgical training and academic leadership from 1994 to 2015. Am J Surg 2016;212(4):566–72.e1.

26. Valsangkar N, Fecher AM, Rozycki GS, et al. Understanding the Barriers to Hiring and Promoting Women in Surgical Subspecialties. J Am Coll Surg 2016;223:387–98.e2.

27. Williams KM, Wang H, Bajaj SS, et al. Career Progression and Research Productivity of Women in Academic Cardiothoracic Surgery. Ann Thorac Surg 2022. https://doi.org/10.1016/j.athoracsur.2022.04.057.

28. Van Doren S, Brida M, Gatzoulis MA, et al. Sex differences in publication volume and quality in congenital heart disease: Are women disadvantaged? Open Heart 2019;6(1). https://doi.org/10.1136/openhrt-2018-000882.

29. Jagsi R, Guancial EA, Worobey CC, et al. The "gender gap" in authorship of academic medical literature–a 35-year perspective. N Engl J Med 2006;355(3):281–7.

30. Eloy JA, Svider P, Chandrasekhar SS, et al. Gender disparities in scholarly productivity within academic otolaryngology departments. Otolaryngol Head Neck Surg 2013;148(2):215–22.

31. Allen I. Women doctors and their careers: What now? BMJ 2005;331(7516):569.

Outside the Operating Room
Alternative Pathways for Doctors and Surgeons to Lead

Robert James Cerfolio, MD, MBA

KEYWORDS

- Leadership • Innovation • Quality efficiency index • Coachability languages

KEY POINTS

- Surgeons make outstanding administrators and leaders.
- Need to learn how to actively listen and make tough decisions.
- Understand why you want to lead, be authentic to yourself.
- Know the different leadership styles, when and how to implement them.
- Know the different coachability languages.
- Know how to leverage quality data (efficiency quality index) to inspire change.

INTRODUCTION

As cardiothoracic surgeons, we spend most of our early childhood and adult lives working, exceeding, and excelling, from grammar school to medical school. Unfortunately, in many situations, we have had to outperform our colleagues in order to achieve one of the few limited positions available. This process influences our mindset and leadership style. In addition, we have had to hone our skills and practiced thousands of hours in the operating room at all hours of the night and on weekends and holidays. We operate and perform under pressure. This process as well forms our personalities. It develops grit, toughness, and forges perseverance. And the very process of our training influences us in many other ways as well.

The journey to become an outstanding technical surgeon and the necessary training improves on our personal attributes and meanwhile may hinder some of our leadership qualities. For example, if the training rewards the few standing, it overtly or subconsciously has us wishing our colleagues to perform worse than we do. This is quite different than outperforming someone who has achieved their best in order for us to reach the next rung on the ladder.

The reality is that other surgeons and physicians and indeed health-care systems are *not* our competition. Rather, they are our colleagues and part of our team. We need all team members of the team to achieve their highest level in order for all of us to reach our full potential as individuals and as a collective team. This concept of team outcomes is leadership. We believe that leaders make everyone around them better. A Schadenfreude mind-set is not part of a winning team. This type of culture was created in part by the old pyramidal training programs that too many of us trained under as opposed to our current training paradigm. It was and is a major obstacle that many surgeons must overcome in order to lead effectively. The best leaders uplift their colleagues and improve their outcomes while simultaneously improving their own.

Funding: None.
Department of Cardiothoracic Surgery, NYU Langone, 531 First Avenue, Suite 9V, New York, NY 10016, USA
E-mail address: Robertjcerfolio77@gmail.com

thoracic.theclinics.com

UNDERSTANDING FAILURE

Most surgeons' entire lives have been marked mainly by successes. We do not do well with failure. We are not trained how to accept it or how best to respond to it. We have many courses on how best to treat and diagnose an ailment in a patient but none on how to react when a patient we operate on has a poor outcome or an important-well-to-do patient chooses another surgeon over us. Most of us have had fast ascents through the academic ranks from assistant, to associate, to full professors. Most authors of this issue are divisional chiefs or chairs of departments. Many have held major leadership roles at national and/or international societies and/or hold executive leadership roles in their respective health-care systems. Do these titles make them leaders? Or do leaders get titles?

In this article, I will share my perspective from the C-Suite about leadership from a surgeon's perspective. As an Executive Vice President (EVP) and Chief Operating Officer (COO) of NYU Langone Health and Vice Dean of NYU Langone Medical School for 5 years, I—a word we rarely use in leadership—will provide my perspective of this pathway of leadership, "outside the operating room." Many lessons we have learned from the operating room and the athletic field can be applied in our many leadership roles out of the operating room as well. Moreover, many of our views must be tempered and even reversed 180° in order to be an effective hospital administrator of a large health-care system. This is the challenge we all accept and enjoy as we struggle to super perform in the many roles we play.[1]

VANTAGE POINT

Because leadership is a personal journey, I can best share my own journey. The word I should almost never if ever appear or be spoken in leadership roles unless one is chronicling their own journey as we do in this article. Thus, in a way for this chapter we/I have to break the "I" rule. There are no prospective randomized trials or P values to reference when one is a surgeon or physician and considering a career in the C suite as a hospital administrator. There is no hard science for us to quote or offer. Experiential data is best. Yet, it must be taken with the filter that it is I who provides it. Only your experience truly matters. And thus, this version is biased on all of my own inherent and learned biases. We have learned that no matter the level of bias-training we undergo, bias still exists. I, again a word we rarely if ever use except in an article such as this, am only able to share my

views and perspective and experience based on my filtered view of leadership. Given this backdrop, we will provide a framework to help guide you on your own unique leadership journey that must be authentic to you and built and mapped by you.

CRITICAL QUESTIONS TO ASK

Before choosing any career pathway, you should carefully ask yourself several challenging introspective questions and realize that your answers may change as you grow. Therefore, we must remain dynamic and nimble and flexible in every way. In the contracts we sign, in the homes we build, in the lives of our families around us and in roles we accept at work. We must fully understand the inherent legal and ethical restrictions they contain and the language must be fully understood. Because our wants and desires change as we age. It is best to stay nimble as we age and as our families age and change and move. With this in mind, we must frequently ask ourselves the following:

1. What type of work truly makes me the happiest?
2. What are my ultimate work goals?
3. Why do I want to lead at work?
4. Who or what groups of individuals do I want to lead at work and why them?
5. Do I really want to lead or do I want the title, money, and prestige that come with the role?
6. What type of leadership style will I use most frequently and is that authentic to me?
7. What is the work team's goal?
8. What is my ultimate desired leadership role?
9. How long should this leadership role last?
10. What is my exit strategy going in?
11. What is my personal goal in this work role?
12. If I choose a leadership role outside of the operating room can I see myself as not operating anymore? Will I be happy out of the operating room and seeing patients all together?
13. What is the team's ultimate goal academically and financially?
14. Who are the members of the team that I lead and do I want to lead them in the culture the role provides? Can I change the culture?

THE WHY

The most important questions to ask yourself are the first 3 above. What makes you the happiest? Why do you want the leadership role and why were you offered it? Why do you want to be an administrator and is it full-time? Can you operate and/or do you want to? Often times, surgeons choose an administrative pathway because of health reasons or because they technically have struggled or current struggle in the operating room either physically or mentally. Or they need a new challenge or problem set. Do you still enjoy operating? Be honest with yourself. This will help you immensely in defining your new role.

When I was first offered the EVP and COO job, I was told that I could not operate, and I declined. Not operating at 54 years of age was not an option for me. At that time, I saw myself first as a surgeon and enjoyed the art of surgery and teaching. What about you? When asked "What do you do for a living—how do you answer and why? How do you see yourself? When and where are you the happiest? For me, the answer was in the operating room. I still loved then and now the operating room and am often the happiest on operative days sitting on the robotic console digging out the pulmonary artery and removing lung cancer.

There is a growing thought that effective administrators should not participate in patient care. Patients care is a 24-hour a day job and when a patient is sick and needs you, their doctor, you cannot be unavailable because you have a meeting. Doctors that miss meetings are ineffective administrators. This is why many doctors that are hospital administrators are not busy surgeons or perform complex high-risk surgery such as cardiothoracic surgeons. Performing the 2 roles concomitantly is difficult, and hence this mindset from administrators that practicing doctors make poor administrators and visa-versa.

The other side of the argument is that all administrators that run hospitals should be a doctor and all should continue to practice medicine to some degree. As your roles increase in an organization, your time spent as a practicing doctor decrease. But those that argue this side suggest it should not be eliminated. Their reason is that the doctor's world changes rapidly. The leader of an organization that loses touch of that world quickly becomes ineffective and not well respected. They believe that there is no better way to truly understand the workforce you serve, the problems they experience and the cultural they work in then to see it for yourself. Just because you used to practice years ago does *not* make you a good administrator now. You are not as well respected as one who does it currently and does it well. Practicing medicine forces you to work in the hospital you run. Visiting every unit in the hospital as an administrator dressed in a suit on leadership rounds with a large group of people who report to you is not the same as having patients there and seeing how it really runs. This debate will continue.

What Makes You the Happiest/Mentoring?

If you truly enjoy teaching and serving medical students, residents, fellows, and patients and families, can you do this in your new job? We had many administrative fellows. My love language is service, what is yours? Can you serve and be faithful to your authentic love and work language as your lead? I declined the role unless I could still operate at least 2 days a week and that is what I did for 5 years while serving as COO and EVP. It was the best decision I ever made. First, it made me a much more effective and respected leader. It provides great "street-cred" when you challenge other practicing physicians to improve their quality metrics such as length of stay, 30-day and 90-day mortalities, discharge before 10 AM, major morbidity, readmissions rate, patient and family satisfaction scores, seeing new patients within 24 hours, returning patients requests in Epic within 24 hours, teaching scores, operative dictation performed within 24 hours, and hospital-acquired conditions. There is no better way to ask others to change and improve than to model the behavior in your own practice. If you can do it, it is easier to ask others to do it as well. This type of leadership that many (too many) surgeons use is called pacesetting leadership. It is usually neither the optimal type of leadership nor a scalable type of leadership style. However, similar to any leadership style, at times, it is effective and you need to know them all and know when to use them all. If you do decide to lead outside the operating room, you will need to add a few other skills to your own toolbox as well.

REQUIRED SKILLS TO LEAD OUTSIDE OF THE OPERATING ROOM
Active Listening and the Leadership Styles

There are 2 critical skills required to succeed as an administrator that we, as surgeons, do not traditionally hone. The first is active listening. The second is how and when to leverage the different leadership styles.

As surgeons, we are taught to act and to act quickly and decisively based on the data given to us. Most often our decisions are fast and definitive and made by you and you alone. We as surgeons are great at this. Who is ready to give their order at a restaurant sooner than a surgeon? In leadership out of the operating room, the exact opposite skill set is needed. Active listening in long meetings that occur all day every day is needed. You must actively listen for long periods without interjecting any bias in your thoughts, and it is best not to speak at all. All team members must feel valued and heard. Most of your team members will be older than you and more experienced than you in their scope of work (pharmacy, pediatrics, food and other ancillary services, regulations and regulatory bodies, infrastructure and engineering, real estate and development, contract negotiations with the third-party payers, philanthropy and complex hospital finances, to name just a few). Your job as their leader is to ensure they achieve their best outcomes and thus maximize your team's value. This only occurs if you listen more then you talk and you ask the right questions.

Understanding of the Different Leadership Styles

Most authors on leadership cite or list 6 major leadership styles. These are as follows: [2]

1. Coercive
2. Authoritative
3. Affiliative
4. Democratic
5. Pace-setting
6. Coaching

During the past several years, there has been a proliferation of listed or cited leadership styles, including transformative, delegative, transactional, servant, participative, and so forth. Despite popular belief, there is no optimal style. Too often experts' cite affiliative as the optimal leadership style. Affiliate leaders often receive the highest scores on 360 surveys and have many advantages but, too often, they do not optimize performance or executive outcomes. At the end of the day, outcomes are our most important metrics as administrators. We must maximize these in order to serve the staff we serve. Other critical metrics are culture assessment and employment engagement scores.

In general, there is no best or optimal leadership style. The best leaders possess the ability to use all of the leadership styles at all time. They have them all at their fingertip and in their toolbox. They know when to use one over another and often implement several of them simultaneously. Moreover, within each style is a multitude of nuances and variances. Over time and with experience great leaders understand their team and the different culture among their team members and know best when to implement one style over another. They also know their own authentic style and remain true to themselves.

More importantly although and unfortunately less cited or understood is that leaders must know which style works best for which team member. Effective leaders understand the "coachability language" [3] of each team member and appropriately use this information to obtain the best out of each individual and their team as a whole. We have studied this and have published on the 8 coachability languages.

The 8 coachability languages that mentees best respond to are as follows:

1. Words of praise
2. A challenge or competition
3. Evidence-base data, informatics, and metrics
4. Coach/mentor's disappointment
5. Team's reliance on their individual role
6. Pride/accomplishments of causes larger than themselves
7. Physical praise (pat on the back)
8. Hardware or money, status, or titles

Similar to leadership styles or love languages no one is only one or the other. Most of us respond to all of these but may respond *best* to one coachability style over another. Over time, a leader must learn their team member and know their coachability language. They must also model this to their direct reports and then inculcate these principals so that their reports will teach it and inculcate it in their own interaction with their direct reports, and so and so on. In this way, one leader can effectively influence the entire culture of a large organization. We do recommend that occasionally you dive down 2 or even 3 levels and meet with some of those reports. However, in general, you have to trust them your direct reports to foster "your culture" downward into the organization and instill it.

We are often asked if a Master of Business Administrative degree or a Master of Public Health or a Master of Health Care Administrative Degree is needed to be an effective leader. These degrees and/or additional training such as them are helpful. They may also help you learn the language of administrators and of the pecuniary world of hospitals. However, a few letters at the end of your name is not a replacement for carefully mastering the nuances of listening, creating a safe space to innovate and fail and to fully understand and practice executive leadership.

IMPACT

If your interest in administration is making a greater influence on the lives of more people around you than you can as a surgeon, we share goals. This was the main reason I went into administration. I thought I could influence the lives of more people as an administrator than as a surgeon no matter how many operations I performed or how many partners we hired. I wanted to have a larger influence on the doctors' and nurses' and staff members' lives. I heard their complaints every day and knew we could do better. The influence that each one of us makes on those around is perhaps the most important part of what we leave behind. This is our legacy. It is shaped by our character. It is marked by how we treat others and the processes that we improve and implement in order to make their lives better and the lives of the patients we serve better.

We cannot institute change unless we inspire others to care for their patients better. Perhaps, the largest challenge that continues to haunt administrators is they present doctors with data that are either wrong or measure the wrong metrics or worse—both. For these reasons, we have created the efficiency quality index (EQI) and we believe it is the single most important reason for the vast improvement that we have enjoyed in the US News and World ranking from 32 to 3.

THE EFFICIENCY QUALITY INDEX

Dash boards and real-time data is the only way to inspire improvement. We, as administrators, too often present data that are old, not actionable, measure the wrong metrics, or worse contain data that are just inaccurate. Then when busy physicians question it, too many administrators still fail to understand the differences in physicians' practices or how to account risk-adjusted data to make comparisons fair.[4] Once you have presented a doctor with data that are wrong, you have lost their heart for years if not forever. For this reason, you cannot present poor data to your staff.

We innovated and created a new metric that accurate measures quality and efficiency. It is called The EQI,[5] which provides a score for each specific operation and/or the care of one specific conditions. We have used the EQI for hospitalists, surgeons, infectious disease physicians, and for staff members. You must ensure that you compare apples to apples only and then guard against poor performers from public embarrassment or feeling devalued. The goal is not to just celebrate the best performers but to have them share best of practice and improve the performance of everyone, especially the bottom 20%. The EQI only measures metrics of quality outcomes that doctors decide are the optimal surrogates of quality for each operation. Thus, the physician cannot say that the wrong metrics were measured because they decided what to measure. Moreover, they cannot state the data are wrong because The EQI only cites and the leverages accurate data that are vetted by each doctor and then approved by the doctors before the EQI is tabulated.[6] It affords fair comparisons, and once egos are set aside, the EQI quickly improves care to all patients because the optimal patient care plan is implemented by everyone, eventually.

CLINICS CARE POINTS

None for this article.

ACKNOWLEDGMENTS

None.

DISCLOSURE

None—all conflicts of interest were removed and have kept as such—while served as EVP, COO, and Vice Dean. The author has nothing to disclose.

DECLARATION OF INTERESTS

None.

REFERENCES

1. Cerfolio R, James Super Performing at Work and Home. The athleticism of surgery and life. Austin Tx: River Gross Books; 2013.
2. Cerfolio, Robert J Cerfolio. Inspire, Available at: www.ICGGtesting.com. Printed in USA LCCN: 2017962940.
3. Cerfolio RJ, Ferrari Light D. How to get the most out of your trainees in robotic thoracic surgery-"the coach-ability languages ". Ann Cardiothorac Surg 2019;8: 269–73.
4. Cerfolio RJ, Commentary. Scrubs united with suits to provide quality care and profits. J Thorac Cardiovasc Surg 2023;166(3):699–700.
5. Cerfolio RJ, Chang SH. Efficiency Quality Index (EQI) – Implementing a novel metric that delivers overall institutional excellence and values for patients. Front Surg 2021;Feb 1:7"604916.
6. Cerfolio RJ. Resistance to change from Super performers: The EQI, Ego and the Safety Card. Ann Thor Surg 2022;Sep 14:S0003–4975.

Implementation of Well-Being for Cardiothoracic Surgeons

Sarah Khalil, MD[a], Anna Olds, MD[b], Kristine Chin, BS[c], Cherie P. Erkmen, MD[d],*

KEYWORDS

- Well-being • Wellness • Thoracic surgery • Cardiothoracic surgery • Residency • Faculty • Burnout

KEY POINTS

- Burnout has three dimensions: (1) mental and/or physical exhaustion; (2) depersonalization, disconnection, negativism, or cynicism related to one's job; (3) reduced professional efficacy.
- Six core principles of well-being: (1) progress toward a goal; (2) actions commensurate with experience, interest, mission; (3) interconnectivity with others; (4) social relatedness; (5) safety; and (6) autonomy.
- Prioritize actions that fulfill the core principles of well-being and avoid/expeditiously complete actions that do not contribute to well-being.
- Like the skills of surgery, skills of mindfulness, resilience, and connection with others must be practiced.
- Well-being among individuals cannot be achieved without support of workplace leaders and durable institutional infrastructure.

WELL-BEING

Well-being is a growing priority in cardiothoracic surgery and across medicine. The Accreditation Council for Graduate Medical Education has prioritized "well-being" in the training environment and established requirements and responsibilities for training institutions to integrate into the learning environment. Cardiothoracic-specific well-being guidelines for programs have been identified,[1] and a checklist for integration of well-being into Thoracic Surgery Training Programs is available[2] to program directors and trainees. The Thoracic Surgery Directors Association and the Thoracic Surgery Resident's Association have collaborated to develop Web-based educational content[3] on well-being. The Association for Academic Thoracic Surgeons (AATS) has a well-being workforce that produces sessions in the AATS Annual Meeting, webinars, collaborative meetings, and research in well-being among cardiothoracic surgeons. Furthermore, the Society of Thoracic Surgeons (STS) has addressed well-being within its workforce on early practice.[1,4] Despite a concerted effort by multiple organizations, our field has yet to develop comprehensive best practices that integrate well-being into thoracic surgery practice. Cardiothoracic surgeons are critically important to medical institutions, both in the service they provide and profit margins.[5] With the expected shortage of cardiothoracic surgeons,[6] we cannot afford to lose any of our highly skilled colleagues to burnout.

[a] Department of General Surgery, Western Michigan University, Homer Stryker MD School of Medicine, 1000 Oakland Drive, Kalamazoo, MI 49008, USA; [b] Division of Cardiac Surgery, Department of Surgery, Keck School of Medicine of USC, University of Southern California, 1520 San Pablo Street, Suite 4300, Los Angeles, CA 90033, USA; [c] Lewis Katz School of Medicine at Temple University, 3500 North Broad Street, Philadelphia, PA 19140, USA; [d] Department of Thoracic Medicine and Surgery, Lewis Katz School of Medicine at Temple University, 3401 North Broad Street, Suite 501, Parkinson Pavilion, Philadelphia, PA 19140, USA
* Corresponding author.
E-mail address: Cherie.p.erkmen@tuhs.temple.edu

Thorac Surg Clin 34 (2024) 63–76
https://doi.org/10.1016/j.thorsurg.2023.08.006
1547-4127/24/© 2023 Elsevier Inc. All rights reserved.

Well-being on a cardiothoracic surgery team is difficult to define, evaluate, and manage. Brady and colleagues defined physician well-being as quality of life with positive physical, mental, social, and integrated experience in connection with activities and environments that allow physicians to develop their full potential across personal and work–life domains.[7] Although many physicians may seek time away from work to achieve well-being, thoracic surgeons may derive well-being from the workplace, in the operating room, and with patients, trainees, and colleagues. In addition, cardiothoracic surgeons, who are sufficiently driven and resilient to handle the rigors of cardiothoracic training and practice, may not benefit from general well-being training.[1,8] Cardiothoracic surgeons may find greater benefit from specialty-specific training in burnout prevention, resilience with care of high-risk patients, institutionally supported strategies to optimize efficiency or personnel to assist with administrative work that cardiothoracic surgeons may not enjoy. Well-being as a physical, mental, social, and integrated experience is a dynamic definition that changes from person to person, and well-being for an individual may change with environments or over time. Intersectional factors of gender, race, and ethnicity can further impact well-being and the ability to manage burnout symptoms. Despite the individual nature of well-being, evidence demonstrates that group, institutional, and environmental factors directly impact well-being.[9] Thus, it is the responsibility of all (individuals, sections, divisions, departments, and institutions) to invest in durable infrastructure to preserve well-being.

BURNOUT

The World Health Organization classifies burnout as an occupational phenomenon resulting from chronic workplace stress.[10] Burnout has three dimensions: (1) a state of energy depletion, mental and/or physical exhaustion; (2) depersonalization, increased mental distance from one's job, or feelings of negativism or cynicism related to one's job; and (3) reduced professional efficacy. Burnout includes illness and injury that result from chronic stress[11] (**Fig. 1**). In the medical setting, burnout is associated with increased medical errors, lack of professionalism, adverse patient outcomes, low patient satisfaction, and increased medical malpractice suits.[1,12–16] Burnout is also related to compassion fatigue,[17] a detachment from the caring about others' suffering. Instead of gaining happiness and value from patient interactions, physicians may feel burdened, irritable, intolerant, or cynical when caring for patients. Burnout is associated with threefold[18] increase in intention to quit working. Early career physicians were especially prone to burnout.

The COVID-19 pandemic demonstrated how stress from inside and outside the workplace can impact burnout. Before the COVID-19 pandemic, the prevalence of burnout among surgeons was 34% and 51% among residents.[19,20] Forty-three percent of surgical residents experienced weekly burnout symptoms with higher burnout symptoms associated with attrition and suicidal thoughts.[21] The pandemic led to increased burnout, depression, and dissatisfaction with quality of life among health care workers.[9,12] During the height of the pandemic, women and minorities were reported to have stress and burnout symptoms higher than the general population.[22] Women were found to have a greater rate of unemployment, increased domestic work, and more childcare responsibilities than men, leading to increased mental health problems.[22,23] Households containing a minority member were more likely to report a decline in total income during the pandemic, adding an additional level of stress to household well-being.[22] A survey conducted by the wellness committee of the AATS in 2021 after the second wave of the COVID-19 pandemic found that among 871 cardiothoracic surgeons and trainees interviewed, many experienced moderate signs of burnout. These included a sense of dread and emotional exhaustion.[24] In addition, most respondents indicated that they had no resources to help them manage their burnout symptoms.[24]

The purpose of this work is to develop evidence-based guidelines promoting well-being in thoracic surgery, at individual and institutional levels. With these guidelines, our goal is to guide implementation of sustainable well-being practices.

We focus on six core principles of well-being as they relate to work–life integration.

1. Making progress toward a goal
2. Actions that are commensurate with experience, interest, and mission
3. Interconnectivity with others
4. Social relatedness to the work that we do
5. Safety
6. Autonomy

Each of these principles foster motivation and the ability to derive meaning from an integrated work–life of a cardiothoracic surgeon. Actions that align with these principles are likely to increase well-being, gratefulness, motivation, and energy to propel productivity. Actions that do not align with principles may be necessary but should be minimized, deprioritized, and completed

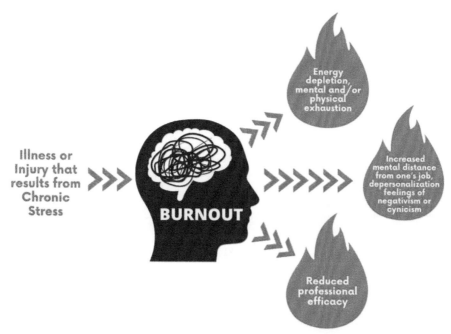

Fig. 1. Dimensions of burnout. (*Adapted from* Pai P et al. Health Serv. 2022;2:844305.)

expeditiously. **Fig. 2** shows a summary of the six principles and strategies to achieve them.

MAKING PROGRESS TOWARD A GOAL

A strong sense of personal accomplishment improves well-being and is protective against burnout.[25] Trainees have measurable annual milestones of progressing to graduation. Measurable goals for faculty and practicing surgeons are more difficult to define. Accomplishment can be in the form of mastery of operative abilities, acquiring a new technique, achieving benchmarks of volume or quality, academic contribution such as publication or presentation, inclusion among a group like STS and AATS membership, or a leadership position. The COVID-19 pandemic limited case volumes, drastically changed patient care opportunities, canceled society meetings, and stalled leadership and promotion, thus diminishing opportunities for accomplishment and motivation among cardiothoracic surgeons and trainees. A decrease in operative experience among surveyed plastic surgery trainees resulted in a reported negative effect on education in greater than 50%, and a negative effect on well-being in more than 80%.[26] This drop in case volume is not unique to plastic surgery and was demonstrable across all case types in general surgery resident case logs.[27] Concerns expressed by trainees about inability to meet case logs due to redeployment and decrease in case volumes also increased burnout symptoms throughout surgical trainees in

multiple specialties.[28] It is unknown how these gaps in training will impact cardiothoracic surgeons in the future. However, it is likely that cardiothoracic surgeons will feel added uncertainty if not anxiety about their preparation for practice in the future. Case volume also impacts practicing surgeons. With a decrease in volume or hiatus in care, even routine cases become challenging. This may be a result of surgeon practice but also a result of changes in qualified personnel within the team, team dynamics, equipment, or available supplies. Supply and staffing shortages can lead to increased difficulty both in the operating room and in the perioperative care of patients.

Setting challenging, specific, and achievable goals is one of the best-established tools to increase performance, motivation, and productivity in a workplace. The achievement of these goals leads to increased perception of success and greater self-esteem.[29] Failing to achieve high and specific goals leads to increased absenteeism, negative responses to experiences, and increased burnout.[29,30] Goal revision is one way to combat failure, as is setting smaller goals that are attainable while building to achieve a larger goal.[29] Successful individuals share the common behavior of believing in their ability to achieve goals, adapting to changing environments, and revising goals accordingly.[31] Setting and achieving attainable goals with the ability to revise these goals over time leads to increased satisfaction with work, decreased burnout, and improved well-being.[32]

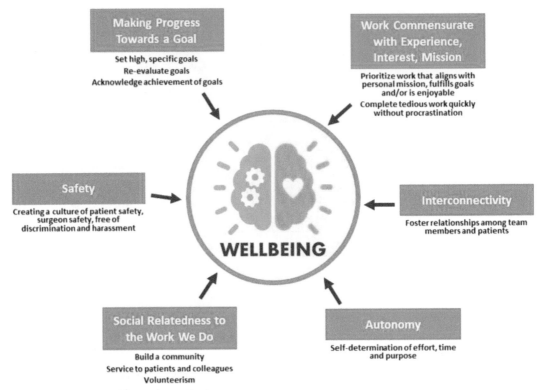

Fig. 2. Principles of well-being for cardiothoracic surgeons.

Goal setting applies to individuals but also clinical/research teams, practices, departments, and institutions. Goal setting is fundamental to successful management of health care institutions. Ogbeiwi reviewed goal setting in organizational management and found that goal setting can effectively motivate attainment if using the Specific, Measurable, Achievable, Relevant/Realistic and Timely/Time-bound framework.[33] Goals may reflect patient volume, quality of care delivered, or academic/administrative expectations. Goals should be problem-based and change-oriented. Goals must be refreshed and adapted to the current context. For example, a shortage of personnel may begin as a goal to recruit qualified team members but change to a goal of training personnel with potential. Acknowledging success and congratulating oneself are also a practice of wellness.[34] Positive reinforcement and self-talk have been shown to impact physiology of pain and weight loss as well as performance among students and athletes.[35–38] Leveraging reflections of previous accomplishments, people can positively influence goal setting, believing in oneself, and perhaps even performance. Neglecting accomplishments and negative self-talk can prevent people from setting goals and discourage effort. Whether at the individual or institutional level,

strategic and frequent goal setting and acknowledgment of achievement can improve well-being of cardiothoracic surgeons.

WORK THAT IS COMMENSURATE WITH EXPERIENCE, INTEREST, AND MISSION

Another principle of well-being is devoting effort to work that aligns with experience, interest, and personal mission. Cardiothoracic surgeons have received in-depth and specific training for cardiothoracic diseases. Duties or work outside the scope of training can result in stress and frustration. During the COVID-19 pandemic, many cardiothoracic surgeons and trainees were assigned to responsibilities outside of their usual practice.[28] Staffing shortages amid COVID-19 also resulted in cardiothoracic surgeons assuming clerical, nursing, or support responsibilities. Even work within the scope of practice, such as peer-to-pear meetings with insurance providers and medical documentation, is frequently cited as a source of burnout. Administrative and clerical tasks adversely affect physicians' ability to deliver high-quality care.[39] Information technology-related stress independently predicts burnouts among physicians.[40,41] However, physician-driven solutions such as scribes and user-friendly electronic medical record interfaces can improve physician well-being. These measures have also been shown to increase productivity and favorable interactions with patients, further enhancing well-being for physicians.[42] Structural workflow and personnel changes that relieve physicians from tedious, frustrating, or nonclinical tasks require buy-in from leadership. Institutions and leaders can advance wellness by valuing cardiothoracic surgeons and prioritizing their desire to care for patients and operate.

Those in leadership positions should recognize that requiring individuals to do unfamiliar or undesirable work is especially harmful to well-being. Work that does not contribute to an individual's well-being or advancement, but benefits the organization has been termed, "office housework."[43] For example, serving on hospital committees, educating nurses and allied professionals, and developing quality initiatives may benefit the group, but they require time and work of the cardiothoracic surgeon that is often not compensated. Furthermore, if these responsibilities are not of interest to the individual being tasked with the job, the cardiothoracic surgeon's well-being will suffer. The individual cardiothoracic surgeon must advocate for himself/herself to decline or limit responsibilities that will detract from well-being. If it is not possible to decline unwanted responsibilities, then the individual should limit time effort invested in the unfavored tasks. Timely completion of unwanted tasks will help well-being by limiting the duration of worry or frustration. Those in leadership position should identify "office housework," match it with individuals who may be find value in some responsibilities and equitably distribute it among partners. Those tasked with "office housework" should be compensated for their time and work. Investment in efficient infrastructure and personnel to help cardiothoracic surgeons will be less than the cost of burnout among cardiothoracic surgeons.

Cardiothoracic surgeons can foster their own well-being by recognizing purpose and gratitude in what they do. Cardiothoracic surgeons are dedicated to working stressful, long hours, sometimes at the sacrifice of their own well-being. However, all work is not equal. Some work is valuable, fulfilling, and easy, whereas other work is trivial, tedious, and burdensome. To approach work from a wellness standpoint, individuals should define personal missions and goals. Cardiothoracic surgeons must purposely appreciate work that aligns with personal missions, fulfills goals, and/or provides enjoyment. Acknowledging gratitude, specifically the privilege of being a cardiothoracic surgeon, fosters humility and goodwill

that benefits the cardiothoracic surgeon, the patient, and others in the care environment.[44] The medical paradigm is to identify and focus on pathology and neglect well-being. A positively guided paradigm may improve well-being of patients and cardiothoracic surgeons. Interventions of gratitude training among health care workers improved job satisfaction, teamwork, dedication to the job, and decreased absences from work.[45–47] Gratitude does not imply that cardiothoracic surgeons should be content or normalizing distress. Gratitude can coexist with ambition to change oneself or work environments that are suboptimal. However, a practice of gratitude can give perspective of "building what is strong" instead of focusing on "when things go wrong."[48] All work cannot be interesting or directly related to a meaningful purpose. Work that is necessary but tedious should be done immediately, so that procrastination does not add to the burden. As mentioned previously, because cardiothoracic surgeons are valuable to institutions, leaders in health care should invest in the well-being of cardiothoracic surgeons and minimize work that cardiothoracic surgeons identify as tedious.

INTERCONNECTIVITY WITH TEAM MEMBERS AND PATIENTS

Productive work environments depend on healthy relationships of team members within the workplace. Workplace cooperation can deepen problem-solving, efficiency of work, and lasting engagement of team members. Having a continuity of effort among team members adds commitment and meaning to the work.[49] People reporting high levels of social support in the workplace have fewer claims of disability and absenteeism.[50] Individuals experiencing isolation and lack of community are at high risk of burnout.[49,51,52] Care must be taken to limit duties that isolate individuals from their colleagues or remove them from their usual environment.

Disagreement among team members has only been exacerbated by the barriers to communication imposed by the pandemic. Most of the health care workers experience conflict in the workplace as frequently as weekly.[53] A negative association between group conflict and employee performance has been demonstrated throughout workplace environments.[54] Differences in personal and political beliefs can also contribute to increased team conflict. It has been shown that differences in political beliefs among physicians lead to different types of care provided.[55] Although not directly studied among health care teams, political differences and disagreements among team members can put stress on the work that a team achieves and the relationships between team members in achieving shared goals. Fostering team building and creating a collaborative team dynamic can lead to better team performance and increased perceived well-being by team members. Well-being within the collaborative environment of cardiothoracic surgery should therefore incorporate principles of healthy team communication and collaboration. Team leaders should seek strategies to mitigate team conflict and optimize well-being.

Connections with patients are some of the most rewarding relationships among cardiothoracic surgeons. Interpersonal communication has certainly been influenced by the pandemic by placing barriers to communication, including masking, virtual meetings, and canceling of meetings. Fifty-five percent of our communication is conveyed by facial expression.[56] Facial coverings, though intended to decrease the risk of COVID transmission, inevitably limit the breadth and depth of communication. Face coverings limit the conveyance of emotions, with all their subtleties. Although the incorporation of telemedicine into the care of patients during the pandemic is a tool that improves on what would otherwise be nonexistent care, it has its own limitations. Practically, telemedicine does not allow the clinician to shake hands, convey comfort though touch, or perform a physical examination. Technical issues are a consistent challenge for patients and providers alike. Cardiothoracic surgeons should prioritize development of relationships with patients as these personal connections directly influence well-being.

SOCIAL RELATEDNESS TO THE WORK THAT WE DO

Building a community contributes to well-being among cardiothoracic surgeons. Participation in regional and national meetings allows for collaboration, sharing ideas, and innovation. Connection to multiple surgeons also fosters collegial and mentorship relationships. Mentorship has been shown to enhance performance, improve learning, and encourage collaboration, furthering well-being of the mentee.[57] Mentors can help mentees build and sustain a successful career,[57] by sharing advice based on an experience of their own success and failures. Mentors themselves derive benefits of reflection, self-awareness, empathy, and interpersonal connection to colleagues.[58] Healthy mentorship relationships protect against burnout and improve emotional intelligence by providing

perspective and support.[52,59] Unfortunately, mentorship has been shown to be lacking among training programs nationwide, especially for women and minorities underrepresented in medicine.[4] To promote well-being, cardiothoracic surgeons should prioritize building a community of mentors, mentees, and peers.

Well-being among cardiothoracic surgeons can also be enhanced through service. Within each institution, surgeons can participate in hospital committees and leadership. This type of service develops knowledge, understanding, and empathy of others in the workplace. This perspective gives a sense of community and value to the effort that one expends in the workplace. Serving as part of hospital leadership also gives cardiothoracic surgeons an opportunity to advocate for well-being policies and well-being among surgeons and other team members. Among residents, participation in well-being committees that focused on engagement, mindfulness events, and advocacy led to greater perceived well-being.[60] Among anesthesia residents, it was shown that mere participation in well-being meetings and interventions significantly decreased burnout and improved well-being.[61] Although participation in hospital committees incurs additional responsibilities, for many, there is well-being value in that this work has the potential to positively influence many colleagues.

Social relatedness to the work of cardiothoracic surgeons includes service to patient communities. Many cardiothoracic surgeons participate in patient advocacy organizations and nonprofit organizations related to the diseases that they treat (the American Heart Association, the American Lung Association, and the American Cancer Society). Cardiothoracic surgeons also find meaning in providing global medical care.[62] Fifty-six non-government organizations provide cardiothoracic services to low-income and middle-income countries.[63] Cardiothoracic surgeons can also provide advocacy for patients and health care professionals by interacting with government agencies regarding health policies and reimbursement.[64,65] Cultivating a social relatedness to work can add value to the work, inspire energy, and improve well-being.

SAFETY

Safety of both the patients and the cardiothoracic work environment impact and are impacted by surgeon well-being. A correlation has been shown between physician burnout and poorer patient safety.[16] This is particularly true in surgeons, in whom burnout confers a 2.5-fold increase of medical error.[16] In turn, patient outcomes are intimately related to a surgeon's reputation, value to their institution, and perhaps even self-worth. Favorable patient outcomes can give meaning to the hard work and stress of caring for a surgical patient. A high volume of successful surgeries is a measure of a surgeon's competence and value. Adverse outcomes negatively impact well-being. Sadness, guilt, and shame from a complication can distract surgeons from their professional and home responsibilities.[66] A complication of a patient may result in investigations, peer review, and litigation. These processes can be isolating and punitive, further impacting well-being. A dangerous spiral between burnout and poor patient outcomes can ensue. Cardiothoracic surgeons, especially those in leadership positions, are responsible for creating a culture that discourages singling out colleagues and trainees when mistakes are made. They are also responsible for providing suitable supervision for trainees and junior partners, particularly coming out of the COVID era.[67] A culture of well-being must include keeping not only patients safe but also colleagues.

Safety of the surgical environment also impacts surgeon well-being. A review by Dairywala and colleagues found that 66% to 94% of surgeons have work-related musculoskeletal pain and 60% have had neck pain within the past 12 months.[68] Thoracic subspecialties that integrate laparoscopic and thoracoscopic techniques have increased the risk of neck, hand, wrist, and arm injuries because of the repetitive and extreme actions needed for handling of instruments and visualizing with video screens. Cardiac surgeons are at significantly higher risk of injuries compared with thoracic surgeons. Cardiac surgeons spend extended periods of time in the same position with the neck flexed to visualize the surgical field. The use of loupes and headlamp increases the load on the cervical spine during surgery.[69] Cardiothoracic surgeons who routinely use fluoroscopy are at an increased risk of injury from bearing additional weight with leaded protection. Unfortunately, surgeons are unlikely to seek care for musculoskeletal pain. Of the 35% of surgeons who did seek help for musculoskeletal pain, 54.5% obtained help from a colleague, 13.6% from their general practitioner, 4.5% from a physiotherapist, 22.7% self-medicated, and 4.5% informed the occupational health.[70] In a survey of 602 cardiothoracic surgeons, Mathey-Andrews found that 64% reported work-related musculoskeletal injuries with 30% requiring time off from work and 20% requiring surgery or the use of narcotics which can impact overall well-being and the ability to function at one's highest potential.[69]

Surgeon well-being can be improved with an intention to optimize physical health in the operating room. Like athletes, surgeons should adhere to stretching, strength training, and cardiovascular fitness. On entering the operating room, surgeons should prioritize positioning of equipment to the benefit of everyone in the room. For example, the operating table height should be at the optimal level of the tallest surgeon with the other surgical team members adapting to the table with standing stools. Lights, video screens, and monitors should be positioned to optimize visualization and minimize musculoskeletal strain. Camera and energy source cords and tubing should be safely secured to prevent tripping of team members. Surgeons take leadership by prioritizing safety measures throughout the case. However, surgeons cannot be solely responsible for safety. Institutions should invest in technology that optimizes ergonomic movement. Although robotic surgery may be a large financial investment, it also facilitates personalized ergonomic movement, which may decrease surgeon injury. Furthermore, institutions should invest in education, prevention, and treatment of work-related injuries. Unfortunately, 90% of cardiothoracic surgeons surveyed believed their institution was not supportive in managing work-related injuries.[69]

Professional safety, the ability to thrive in one's career without bullying, harassment, isolation, or discrimination, also impacts well-being. Harassment and discrimination in surgery are pervasive.[71,72] In a review of 25 studies including 29,980 surgical residents, 63% reported experiencing bullying, 43% experienced discrimination, 29% experienced harassment, and 27% experienced sexual harassment.[73] In a survey of 790 cardiothoracic surgeons, 81% of women and 46% of men had experienced sexual harassment at work. Sources of harassment include surgeons with supervisory or leadership roles, colleagues, and ancillary staff. Unfortunately, 71% did not report actions citing a fear of retaliation with reporting. Although discrimination is unlawful, and bullying and harassment are specifically prohibited by most hospital policies, these actions affect several cardiothoracic surgeons, to the detriment of well-being. The STS has published a consensus statement for approaching these challenges, including action as an individual, as a member of a professional team, and at the national cardiothoracic community level. Cardiothoracic surgeons experiencing bullying, harassment, or discrimination should know that they are not alone. The feeling of isolation can compound any adverse events in one's career. Individual surgeons can also serve as advocates or supporters to anyone who is at risk for harassment or discrimination, including women and those of minority races/ethnicities. At the institutional level, mitigation training regarding bias, harassment, and discrimination must be an iterative process with continued support from leadership. At the national professional level, professional societies should support and disseminate research to assess and mitigate bias, harassment, and discrimination. Creating an environment that allows for open discussions about bias, collaboration and learning are the best way to ensure a culture of well-being among cardiothoracic surgeons.

AUTONOMY

Autonomy is an essential component of well-being. Professionals who have a sense of control over decisions affecting their work have decreased burnout and higher job satisfaction.[74,75] A survey of 582 surgeons found that lack of autonomy or involvement in decisions were associated with burnout and emotional exhaustion.[76] In turn, burnout has been linked to physical, neurologic changes that reduce a physician's sense of control over themselves, and a reduction in connection with others. Arnsten and colleagues found that uncontrollable stress, but not controllable stress, impairs the prefrontal cortex functions of abstract reasoning, higher order decision-making, and resilience.[77] Giving physicians control and autonomy over stressful environments preserves high-level thinking needed to thrive in clinical practice.

Autonomy can be divided into autonomy of effort, time, and goals. How a surgeon allocates effort impacts well-being. Physicians are prepared to devote time and effort to the care of patients. However, the lack of control over effort adversely affects well-being. As mentioned previously, physicians are less likely to have burnout if the time spent working is devoted to meaningful, clinically relevant efforts. To optimize cardiothoracic surgeons' well-being, tasks such as medical documentation and addressing billing inquiries should be delegated to others or optimized. The cardiothoracic surgeon should focus on efforts that no other health professionals can do, such as operating and consulting on surgical patients. This contributes to the cardiothoracic surgeons' well-being but also the institutional efficiency.

Cardiothoracic surgeons are also losing autonomy as mandatory tasks increase. Compliance requirements include but are not limited to continuing medical education, maintaining certifications in professional societies or technical skills, compliance training in safety, Health Insurance Portability and Accountability Act, research practices, or other administrative requirements.[39] Physicians do not have a choice; they must devote effort to these tasks. However, protected administrative time is diminishing among most practices. This loss of autonomy in effort not only impacts well-being in the workplace, but to accomplish them, many physicians must work on personal time, weekends or on vacations. Leadership within organizations that use cardiothoracic surgeons should acknowledge these efforts, organize them for efficient completion, and allow for protected time to complete them.

Current clinical practice has resulted in decreased autonomy regarding time and scheduling. Many cardiothoracic surgeons work for multiple hospitals and clinics. Each location adds complexity to call, clinic, and operating room schedules. Cardiothoracic surgeons must invest time to reconcile the demands of each practice setting, transportation and transition between the settings, and schedules of partners. Cardiothoracic surgeons must be given administrative and clinical support to organize realistic schedules. The recent increase of electronic patient portals, Web-based platforms that allow for remote medical documentation, Web-based meetings, and telemedicine have made physicians more accessible to patients and colleagues. However, few organizations have allocated protected time to manage these increased responsibilities. As a result, personal and free time suffers. Cardiothoracic surgeons must have autonomy to prioritize responsibilities and personal time and create a realistic schedule. Institutions, hospital leadership, and medical culture must acknowledge time commitments, including personal time away from work, and support them accordingly. To do this effectively, organizations must engage the physician workforce in routine assessments of time commitments and autonomy and devise interventions that preserve well-being.

Autonomy in decision-making control over professional and personal goals integrates all aforementioned components of well-being, namely (1) making progress toward a goal; (2) actions that are commensurate with experience, interest, and mission; (3) interconnectivity with others; (4) social relatedness to the work that we do; and (5) safety. Cardiothoracic surgeons should receive support to choose their own clinical, professional, and personal goals. In exercising autonomy in these well-being goals, they are likely to be productive and resilient.

WELLNESS OUTSIDE THE WORKPLACE

Wellness is clearly multifaceted and complex, and it can be difficult to pinpoint specific areas of intervention to address the various aspects of wellness. An important aspect of surgeon wellness encompasses life outside of work. This includes family life, integrating personal life with professional responsibilities, outsourcing tasks at home, having a strong support system, and participating in regular exercise, hobbies, outdoor activities, and organizations outside the workplace. Having these leads to increased satisfaction within the workplace.[78,79] By implementing action plans to address well-being in these categories, we can improve the mental health of our specialty and thereby increase efficiency and professional satisfaction.

Parenthood

We can extrapolate from data gathered in general surgery on topics such as parenthood and surgical training. Several national survey projects have shown significant negative health effects on women surgeons, both in and out of training, who become pregnant or would like to become pregnant.[80] This includes an increased risk of infertility as well as pregnancy complications when compared with women of similar socioeconomic status.[80] In addition to adverse health effects, negative stigma, inadequate maternity leave, and insufficient childcare options contribute to career dissatisfaction and a lack of wellness for women surgical trainees and women surgeons.[80,81] A recent review of literature on motherhood in women surgeons found that maternity leave policies as well as breastfeeding and childcare facilities are inadequate and highly variable between programs.[82] Importantly, many women surgeons in their review agree that greater institutional support would help women surgeons in both their professional and personal well-being.[82] In several studies examining paternity leave trends in general surgery training programs, the investigators concluded that many male residents would prefer more time off and that a cultural shift to support surgical residents becoming parents as a normal part of adult life is necessary.[83,84] There is a significant amount of stigma associated with parental leave for both men and women surgeons, and there are a significant amount of data that would support increased wellness with improved parental support. This comes in the form of parental leave, access to affordable childcare, and a cultural shift away from negative stigma associated with having children as a surgeon.

Childcare

Inadequate access or lack of affordable childcare is often cited as a barrier for surgeon success and a barrier to surgeon well-being.[53–55,57,85,86] Although both genders experience missed work due to lack of childcare, women surgeons are more likely than their male counterparts to miss work.[57] This is another actionable area to improve surgeon wellness and improve professional efficiency. If hospitals provided accessible and affordable childcare for surgeons, including both trainees and attendings, well-being as well as productivity and efficiency would be improved.[58,85] By prioritizing surgeon well-being in the personal realm, professional satisfaction and efficiency would be improved. This is a very tangible way that we can improve cardiothoracic surgeon well-being for both trainees and attendings and continue to recruit the best and brightest to the field.

Association of Women Surgeons Recommendations for Program Support

The Association of Women Surgeons (AWS) published a "Comprehensive Initiative for Healthy Surgical Families During Residency and Fellowship Training" that we can apply for specific suggestions.[85] The first action item is planning for parenthood, where AWS states that trainees should be encouraged to share their plans for parenthood to plan as far in advance as possible. AWS provides suggestions for program directors to support trainees, including working to individualize resident needs and schedules, developing plans, creating a culture of support and inclusivity, improving access to infertility and reproductive treatments, and advocating for mental health needs of trainees.[85] Women surgeons tend to have higher risk pregnancies with a significantly increased risk of complications and thus need personalized and flexible plans to account for their needs. In addition, programs should be providing trainees with information and resources for fertility preservation to increase awareness and accessibility in this high-risk population. Women surgeons miscarry at a significantly higher rate than the general population and must be afforded the time to grieve and maintain personal well-being outside of work.[85]

Home Responsibilities

A survey distributed to male and female orthopedic surgeons with a focus on how surgeons balance home and life responsibilities found that of 377 respondents, women surgeons with or without children performed significantly more household tasks than male surgeons.[87] These tasks included laundry, grocery shopping, and meal preparation. Overall, the study found that women surgeons do significantly more household work than male surgeons.[87] There are opportunities for interception here to improve wellness, in the form of outsourcing tasks such as cleaning, laundry, or repairs. In the study by Higgins and colleagues, female orthopedic surgeons tended to rely significantly more on cleaning and laundry services, whereas male orthopedic surgeons used significantly more outsourced repair services.[87] With less time spent on household duties by outsourcing, surgeons could potentially have a more balanced life with improved well-being. We can apply these concepts to cardiothoracic surgery and use these data for evidence to intervene in these areas.

Another aspect of resilience and personal well-being lies in the relationships we cultivate outside of work. It is important to maintain personal relationships and a support system outside of the professional environment with whom one can share feelings and experiences.[34] An important study surveying significant others (SOs) of cardiothoracic surgeons highlights the negative impact that a career in cardiothoracic surgery can have on home and family life.[88] In the survey, 238 responses were included from SOs of cardiothoracic surgeons. Of these 238 SOs, 66% reported a moderate–severe impact on their family from the stress of their surgeon partner. Furthermore, 63% answered that there was not enough time for family due to their surgeon partner's work demands. This indicates the significant impact that the culture of our field has on personal and home life. In addition, the constant balance of patient care responsibilities, needs of SOs, and the needs of self lead to a feeling of failure and lack of effectiveness as well as emotional exhaustion.[88] The investigators suggest that coaching, counseling, and family support can be important to change the balance of work and home life and to improve emotional resilience.[88] By helping surgeons to balance the needs of work, family and SOs, and self, we can create a more sustainable culture in cardiothoracic surgery.

How to Cultivate Personal Wellness and Resilience

Physical exercise, activities, and hobbies that bring joy outside of work, mindfulness, and meditation practices are preventative and treatment for burnout.[34] Just as the practice of mental exercise has positive influence on well-being, physical exercise has been shown to improve resilience and well-being. Physical exercise should be an integral part of the personal lives of cardiothoracic surgeons.[34] In an important expert review, Maddaus describes the concept of a "resilience bank account" that surgeons can tap into in difficult times.[89] By creating such a repository of skills and coping mechanisms, he argues that surgeons will have an easier time dealing with difficult situations in daily life or larger situations such as malpractice suits or personal devastations. Maddaus's "resilience bank account" is built by focusing on the following: sleep, exercise, mindfulness meditation, gratitude, self-compassion, and compassion toward others.[89] He points out that the same devotion to these habits as the devotion we give to mastering our surgical skills will leave us more capable of tolerating stress, and in an improved state of well-being, both personally and professionally. One review of surgeon burnout and prevention outlines the importance of resilience training for surgeons.[34]

SUMMARY

Principles of well-being among cardiothoracic surgeons include striving toward a goal, work commensurate with goals, interconnectedness with others, social relatedness to work, a culture of safety within a workplace, and autonomy. Life outside the workplace is so much more variable than in the workplace, making well-being principles difficult to circumscribe. However, prioritizing family relationships, family responsibilities, support from communities, activities, exercise, and mindfulness are all known practices of well-being. Well-being is not only an individual responsibility. Clinical and educational organizations, health systems, and professional societies must buy into the culture of wellness. Mission statements and policies must prioritize physician well-being. It is important for all members of a cardiothoracic team to value well-being which will increase productivity, patient safety, and financial health. All members of the team should be accountable for understanding the principles of well-being and adhering to the policies set by the leadership. Cardiothoracic surgery leaders should set an example to trainees and junior partners of incorporating well-being practices into their careers and lives. The implementation of well-being practices should be continually assessed for efficacy. We hope that with these cultural changes, the cardiothoracic workforce will meet the growing demands of patient care and cardiothoracic practice.

CLINICS CARE POINTS

- When screening for burnout, look for evidence of (1) mental and/or physical exhaustion; (2) depersonalization, disconnection, negativism, or cynicism related to one's job; (3) reduced professional efficacy.

- Goal setting at the individual, group, or institutional level can promote well-being when goals are Specific, Measurable, Achievable, Relevant/Realistic, Timely/Time-bound. Work to achieve goals should align with the individual's experience and interest.

- People reporting high levels of social support in the workplace have increased commitment to work and less absenteeism. Individuals experiencing isolation and lack of community are at high risk of burnout. Care must be taken to limit duties that isolate individuals from their colleagues or remove them from supportive social interactions.

- Cardiothoracic surgeons must have a safe environment to practice. A review of optimal ergonomic activities and equipment to support these will reduce pain and injury to surgeons. Professional safety includes an environment that is free of bullying, harassment, isolation, and discrimination. Individuals, leaders, and institutions are responsible for promotion of safe environments for cardiothoracic surgeons.

- Professionals who have a sense of control over decisions affecting their work have decreased burnout and higher job satisfaction. Preserving cardiothoracic surgeons' autonomy of effort, time, and goal will result in greater well-being and productivity.

DISCLOSURE

Authors have nothing to disclose.

REFERENCES

1. Fajardo R, Vaporciyan A, Starnes S, et al. Cardiothoracic surgery wellness: Now and the formidable road ahead. J Thorac Cardiovasc Surg 2020. S0022-5223(20)31409-31414.

2. Fajardo R, Vaporciyan A, Starnes S, et al. Implementation of wellness into a cardiothoracic training program: A checklist for a wellness policy. J Thorac Cardiovasc Surg 2021;161(6):1979–86.

3. Faculty Development Webinars | TSDA https://tsda.org/tsda-meetings/faculty-development-webinars/. Accessed July 15, 2023.

4. Sterbling HM, Molena D, Rao SR, et al. Initial report on young cardiothoracic surgeons' first job: From searching to securing and the gaps in between. J Thorac Cardiovasc Surg 2019; 158(2):632–41.e3.

5. Resnick AS, Corrigan D, Mullen JL, et al. Surgeon contribution to hospital bottom line: not all are created equal. Ann Surg 2005;242(4):530–7 [discussion 537-539].

6. Moffatt-Bruce S, Crestanello J, Way DP, et al. Providing cardiothoracic services in 2035: Signs of trouble ahead. J Thorac Cardiovasc Surg 2018; 155(2):824–9.

7. Brady KJS, Trockel MT, Khan CT, et al. What Do We Mean by Physician Wellness? A Systematic Review of Its Definition and Measurement. Acad Psychiatry J Am Assoc Dir Psychiatr Resid Train Assoc Acad Psychiatry 2018;42(1):94–108.

8. Card AJ. Physician Burnout: Resilience Training is Only Part of the Solution. Ann Fam Med 2018; 16(3):267–70.

9. Rotenstein LS, Torre M, Ramos MA, et al. Prevalence of Burnout Among Physicians: A Systematic Review. JAMA 2018;320(11):1131–50.

10. Burn-out an "occupational phenomenon": International Classification of Diseases. Accessed July 15, 2023. https://www.who.int/news/item/28-05-2019-burn-out-an-occupational-phenomenon-international-classification-of-diseases.

11. Pai P, Olcoń K, Allan J, et al. The SEED Wellness Model: A Workplace Approach to Address Well-being Needs of Healthcare Staff During Crisis and Beyond. Front Health Serv 2022;2:844305.

12. Shanafelt TD, West CP, Dyrbye LN, et al. Changes in Burnout and Satisfaction With Work-Life Integration in Physicians During the First 2 Years of the COVID-19 Pandemic. Mayo Clin Proc 2022;97(12): 2248–58.

13. Halbesleben JRB, Rathert C. Linking physician burnout and patient outcomes: exploring the dyadic relationship between physicians and patients. Health Care Manage Rev 2008;33(1):29–39.

14. Tawfik DS, Profit J, Morgenthaler TI, et al. Physician Burnout, Well-being, and Work Unit Safety Grades in Relationship to Reported Medical Errors. Mayo Clin Proc 2018;93(11):1571–80.

15. Owoc J, Mańczak M, Jabłońska M, et al. Association Between Physician Burnout and Self-reported Errors: Meta-analysis. J Patient Saf 2022;18(1): e180–8.

16. Al-Ghunaim TA, Johnson J, Biyani CS, et al. Surgeon burnout, impact on patient safety and professionalism: A systematic review and meta-analysis. Am J Surg 2022;224(1 Pt A):228–38.

17. Lombardo B, Eyre C. Compassion fatigue: a nurse's primer. Online J Issues Nurs 2011;16(1):3.

18. Hodkinson A, Zhou A, Johnson J, et al. Associations of physician burnout with career engagement and quality of patient care: systematic review and meta-analysis. BMJ 2022;378:e070442.

19. Bartholomew AJ, Houk AK, Pulcrano M, et al. Meta-Analysis of Surgeon Burnout Syndrome and Specialty Differences. J Surg Educ 2018;75(5):1256–63.

20. Low ZX, Yeo KA, Sharma VK, et al. Prevalence of Burnout in Medical and Surgical Residents: A Meta-Analysis. Int J Environ Res Public Health 2019;16(9):1479.

21. Hewitt DB, Ellis RJ, Hu YY, et al. Evaluating the Association of Multiple Burnout Definitions and Thresholds With Prevalence and Outcomes. JAMA Surg 2020;155(11):1043–9.

22. Mejia-Mantilla C. The uneven impact of the pandemic on women and minorities. 2023 https://blogs.worldbank.org/latinamerica/uneven-impact-pandemic-women-and-minorities. Accessed July 15, 2023.

23. COVID-19: Rebuilding for Resilience. UN Women – Headquarters Available at: https://www.unwomen.org/en/hq-complex-page/covid-19-rebuilding-for-resilience. Accessed July 15, 2023.

24. Bremner RM, Ungerleider RM, Ungerleider J, et al. Well-being of Cardiothoracic Surgeons in the Time of COVID-19: A Survey by the Wellness Committee of the American Association for Thoracic Surgery. Semin Thorac Cardiovasc Surg 2022. https://doi.org/10.1053/j.semtcvs.2022.10.002.

25. Khorfan R, Hu YY, Agarwal G, et al. The Role of Personal Accomplishment in General Surgery Resident Well-being. Ann Surg 2021;274(1):12–7.

26. Crowe CS, Lopez J, Morrison SD, et al, Resident Council Wellness and Education Study Group. The Effects of the COVID-19 Pandemic on Resident Education and Wellness: A National Survey of Plastic Surgery Residents. Plast Reconstr Surg 2021;148(3):462e–74e.

27. Purdy AC, de Virgilio C, Kaji AH, et al. Factors associated with general surgery residents' operative experience during the COVID-19 pandemic. JAMA Surg 2021;156(8):767–74.

28. Hope C, Reilly JJ, Griffiths G, et al. The impact of COVID-19 on surgical training: a systematic review. Tech Coloproctology 2021;25(5):505–20 [published correction appears in Tech Coloproctol. 2021 Nov; 25(11):1267-1268].

29. Höpfner J, Keith N. Goal missed, self hit: goal-setting, goal-failure, and their affective, motivational, and behavioral consequences. Front Psychol 2021; 12:704790.

30. Houser-Marko L, Sheldon KM. Eyes on the prize or nose to the grindstone? The effects of level of goal evaluation on mood and motivation. Pers Soc Psychol Bull 2008;34(11):1556–69.

31. Wolf BM, Herrmann M, Brandstätter V. Self-efficacy vs. action orientation: Comparing and contrasting two determinants of goal setting and goal striving. J Res Personal 2018;73:35–45.

32. Shanafelt TD, Noseworthy JH. Executive leadership and physician well-being: nine organizational strategies to promote engagement and reduce burnout. Mayo Clin Proc 2017;92(1):129–46.

33. Ogbeiwi O. General concepts of goals and goal-setting in healthcare: a narrative review. J Manag Organ 2021;27(2):324–41.

34. Naviaux AF, Barbier L, Chopinet S, et al. Ways of preventing surgeon burnout. J Visc Surg 2023; 160(1):33–8.

35. Luo X, Liu J, Che X. Investigating the influence and a potential mechanism of self-compassion on experimental pain: evidence from a compassionate self-talk protocol and heart rate variability. J Pain 2020; 21(7–8):790–7.

36. Browne J, Xie H, Wolfe RS, et al. Factors associated with weight gain prevention in young adults with serious mental illness. Early Interv Psychiatry 2023; 17(1):39–46.

37. Dahl-Leonard K, Hall C, Beegle B, et al. Teaching readers to recognize negative thoughts and use positive self-talk. Interv Sch Clin 2022. https://doi.org/10.1177/10534512221140537. 10534512221140536.

38. Hardy J, Comoutos N, Hatzigeorgiadis A. Reflections on the maturing research literature of self-talk in sport: contextualizing the special issue. Sport Psychol 2018;32(1):1–8.

39. National Academies of Sciences, Engineering, and Medicine; National Academy of Medicine; Committee on Systems Approaches to Improve Patient Care by Supporting Clinician Well-Being. Taking action against clinician burnout: a systems approach to professional well-being. National Academies Press (US); 2019. Available at: http://www.ncbi.nlm.nih.gov/books/NBK552618/. Accessed July 15, 2023.

40. Gardner RL, Cooper E, Haskell J, et al. Physician stress and burnout: the impact of health information technology. J Am Med Inform Assoc JAMIA 2019; 26(2):106–14.

41. Guo U, Chen L, Mehta PH. Electronic health record innovations: helping physicians - One less click at a time. Health Inf Manag J Health Inf Manag Assoc Aust 2017;46(3):140–4.

42. Mishra P, Kiang JC, Grant RW. Association of medical scribes in primary care with physician workflow and patient experience. JAMA Intern Med 2018; 178(11):1467–72.

43. Babcock L, Recalde MP, Vesterlund L, et al. Gender differences in accepting and receiving requests for

tasks with low promotability. Am Econ Rev 2017; 107(3):714–47.

44. Day G, Robert G, Rafferty AM. Gratitude in health care: a meta-narrative review. Qual Health Res 2020;30(14):2303–15.

45. Cheng ST, Tsui PK, Lam JHM. Improving mental health in health care practitioners: randomized controlled trial of a gratitude intervention. J Consult Clin Psychol 2015;83(1):177–86.

46. Stegen A, Wankier J. Generating gratitude in the workplace to improve faculty job satisfaction. J Nurs Educ 2018;57(6):375–8.

47. Burke RJ, Ng ESW, Fiksenbaum L. Virtues, work satisfactions and psychological wellbeing among nurses. Int J Workplace Health Manag 2009;2(3): 202–19.

48. Duckworth AL, Steen TA, Seligman MEP. Positive psychology in clinical practice. Annu Rev Clin Psychol 2005;1:629–51.

49. Kassam A, Horton J, Shoimer I, et al. Predictors of well-being in resident physicians: a descriptive and psychometric study. J Grad Med Educ 2015; 7(1):70–4.

50. White M, Wagner S, Schultz IZ, et al. Modifiable workplace risk factors contributing to workplace absence across health conditions: a stakeholder-centered best-evidence synthesis of systematic reviews. Work Read Mass 2013;45(4):475–92.

51. van Wulfften Palthe ODR, Neuhaus V, Janssen SJ, et al. Ring D, Science of variation group. among musculoskeletal surgeons, job dissatisfaction is associated with burnout. Clin Orthop 2016;474(8): 1857–63.

52. Ishak WW, Lederer S, Mandili C, et al. Burnout during residency training: a literature review. J Grad Med Educ 2009;1(2):236–42.

53. Cullati S, Bochatay N, Maître F, et al. When team conflicts threaten quality of care: a study of health care professionals' experiences and perceptions. Mayo Clin Proc Innov Qual Outcomes 2019;3(1): 43–51.

54. Leon-Perez JM, Antino M, Leon-Rubio JM. The role of psychological capital and intragroup conflict on employees' burnout and quality of service: a multi-level approach. Front Psychol 2016;7:1755.

55. Hersh ED, Goldenberg MN. Democratic and republican physicians provide different care on politicized health issues. Proc Natl Acad Sci U S A 2016; 113(42):11811–6.

56. Mheidly N, Fares MY, Zalzale H, et al. Effect of face masks on interpersonal communication during the COVID-19 Pandemic. Front Public Health 2020;8: 582191.

57. Burgess A, van Diggele C, Mellis C. Mentorship in the health professions: a review. Clin Teach 2018; 15(3):197–202.

58. Henry-Noel N, Bishop M, Gwede CK, et al. Mentorship in medicine and other health professions. J Cancer Educ Off J Am Assoc Cancer Educ 2019;34(4):629–37.

59. Sargent MC, Sotile W, Sotile MO, et al. Stress and coping among orthopaedic surgery residents and faculty. J Bone Joint Surg Am 2004;86(7):1579–86.

60. Tillman F, Behrens A, Moynihan M, et al. Impact of a resident-driven wellbeing committee on resident-perceived wellbeing, burnout, and resilience. J Am Pharm Assoc 2022. S1544-S3191(22)00404-00406.

61. Brainard AJ, Ziniel SI, Zuk J, et al. Evaluation of a formal wellness curriculum to reduce burnout in anesthesia residents: a pilot study. J Educ Perioper Med JEPM 2019;21(1):E631.

62. Mody GN. Global health equity: a vision for engaging thoracic surgeons. Thorac Surg Clin 2022;32(3):xv–xvii.

63. Vervoort D, Guetter CR, Munyaneza F, et al. Non-governmental organizations delivering global cardiac surgical care: a quantitative impact assessment. Semin Thorac Cardiovasc Surg 2022;34(4): 1160–5.

64. Speir AM, Yohe C, Dearani JA. Cardiothoracic surgical advocacy in a time of COVID-19. Ann Thorac Surg 2020;110(4):1101–2.

65. Speir AM, Yohe C, Lahey SJ, et al. STS workforce on health policy, advocacy, and reform, and the workforce on coding and reimbursement. 2020 medicare final payment rule: implications for cardiothoracic surgery. Ann Thorac Surg 2020;109(2):313–6.

66. Srinivasa S, Gurney J, Koea J. Potential consequences of patient complications for surgeon well-being: a systematic review. JAMA Surg 2019; 154(5):451–7.

67. Chaban R, Buschmann K, Dohle DS, et al. Training cardiac surgeons: safety and requirements. Semin Thorac Cardiovasc Surg 2022;34(4):1236–46.

68. Dairywala MI, Gupta S, Salna M, et al. Surgeon strength: ergonomics and strength training in cardiothoracic surgery. Semin Thorac Cardiovasc Surg 2022;34(4):1220–9.

69. Mathey-Andrews C. A National Survey of Occupational Musculoskeletal Injuries in Cardiothoracic Surgeons. Presented at: AATS 103 Annual Meeting; May 2023; Los Angeles, CA Available at: https:// www.aats.org/resources/a-national-survey-of-occupational-musculoskeletal-injuries-in-cardiothoracic-surgeons. Accessed July 15, 2023.

70. Soueid A, Oudit D, Thiagarajah S, et al. The pain of surgery: pain experienced by surgeons while operating. Int J Surg Lond Engl 2010;8(2):118–20.

71. Hu YY, Ellis RJ, Hewitt DB, et al. Discrimination, abuse, harassment, and burnout in surgical residency training. N Engl J Med 2019;381(18): 1741–52.

72. Ceppa DP, Dolejs SC, Boden N, et al. Sexual harassment and cardiothoracic surgery: #UsToo? Ann Thorac Surg 2020;109(4):1283–8.

73. Gianakos AL, Freischlag JA, Mercurio AM, et al. Bullying, discrimination, harassment, sexual harassment, and the fear of retaliation during surgical residency training: a systematic review. World J Surg 2022;46(7):1587–99.

74. Senturk JC, Melnitchouk N. Surgeon burnout: defining, identifying, and addressing the new reality. Clin Colon Rectal Surg 2019;32(6):407–14.

75. Yates SW. Physician stress and burnout. Am J Med 2020;133(2):160–4.

76. Campbell DA, Sonnad SS, Eckhauser FE, et al. Burnout among American surgeons. Surgery 2001; 130(4):696–702. ; discussion 702-705.

77. Arnsten AFT, Shanafelt T. Physician distress and burnout: the neurobiological perspective. Mayo Clin Proc 2021;96(3):763–9.

78. Balch CM, Freischlag JA, Shanafelt TD. Stress and burnout among surgeons: understanding and managing the syndrome and avoiding the adverse consequences. Arch Surg Chic III 1960 2009;144(4): 371–6.

79. Well-Being Concepts | HRQOL | CDC. Published November 5, 2018 https://www.cdc.gov/hrqol/ wellbeing.htm. Accessed July 15, 2023.

80. Rangel EL, Smink DS, Castillo-Angeles M, et al. Pregnancy and motherhood during surgical training. JAMA Surg 2018;153(7):644–52.

81. Rangel EL, Castillo-Angeles M, Easter SR, et al. Incidence of infertility and pregnancy complications in US female surgeons. JAMA Surg 2021;156(10): 905–15.

82. Mavedatnia D, Ardestani S, Zahabi S, et al. The experiences of motherhood in female surgeons: a scoping review. Ann Surg 2023;277(2):214–22.

83. Castillo-Angeles M, Smink DS, Rangel EL. Perspectives of general surgery program directors on paternity leave during surgical training. JAMA Surg 2022; 157(2):105–11.

84. Castillo-Angeles M, Stucke RS, Rosenkranz KM, et al. Paternity leave during surgical training: perspectives of male residents. J Surg Educ 2022; 79(6):e85–91.

85. Johnson HM, Torres MB, Möller MG, et al. Association of women surgeons' comprehensive initiative for healthy surgical families during residency and fellowship training. JAMA Surg 2023;158(3):310–5.

86. Knell J, Kim ES, Rangel EL. The challenges of parenthood for female surgeons: the current landscape and future directions. J Surg Res 2023;288: A1–8.

87. Higgins MJ, Kale NN, Brown SM, et al. Taking family call: understanding how orthopaedic surgeons manage home, family, and life responsibilities. J Am Acad Orthop Surg 2021;29(1):e31–40.

88. Ungerleider JD, Ungerleider RM, James L, et al. Assessment of the well-being of significant others of cardiothoracic surgeons. J Thorac Cardiovasc Surg 2023. https://doi.org/10.1016/j.jtcvs.2023.04. 008. S0022-5223(23)00331-00338.

89. Maddaus M. The resilience bank account: skills for optimal performance. Ann Thorac Surg 2020; 109(1):18–25.

Integrating Advocacy into Your Practice

Keith S. Naunheim, MD*, Joseph J. Platz, MD

KEYWORDS

• Politics • Advocacy • Philanthropy • Ethics • Government • Doctor-patient relationship

KEY POINTS

- Health care has evolved in the last 60 years and the patient-doctor relationship is being impinged upon by government, industry, insurance companies, and health systems.
- Physicians are encouraged to actively participate in advocacy for their patients regarding economic, financial, social, political, and health issues.
- Advocacy can take the form of personal engagement by the physician or via proxy by participation in or support of supporting specialty organizations, charities, nongovernmental organizations, or political causes.

CLASSIC PATIENT-DOCTOR RELATIONSHIP

Delineating the role of the physician in society is a century-old practice, beginning with the Hippocratic Oath in ancient Greece.[1] The concepts of care for all, reverence for one's teachers, proscription from undertaking procedures outside one's expertise, and inviolable confidentiality are all worthy goals. These concepts focus on the clinical care delivered to the patient, primarily on a one-to-one basis, with nary a mention of obligation to individuals other than the patient. This was the health care standard throughout the first 2 centuries of surgical care in the United States. However, soon after World War II, the concept of private health insurance arose and its Implementation began, thus involving the private industry in the previously simple patient-doctor relationship. Soon thereafter, in the 1960s, yet another player entered into this relationship by virtue of legislation passed in President Johnson's Great Society program: the US government. In 1965, the government took a direct role as a third-party payer, reimbursing providers for care to the elderly and disabled via Medicare and for care to the poor via Medicaid. It seemed that the previously simple patient-doctor relationship was now less private and included other parties.

During this same time, we see there was some evolution in the ethical constructs first established by Hippocrates. In 1964, Dr Lasagna aspired to provide an updated version of the physician's oath, including the clause suggesting a physician's responsibility might now extend outside direct patient-doctor relationship.[1]

I will remember that I remain a member of society with special obligations to all my fellow human beings, those sound of mind and body as well as the infirm.

These words suggested for the first time that the ethical duty of the physician should no longer simply be constrained by the classic one-to-one patient-doctor relationship, but rather there existed an obligation to work toward the betterment of society in general outside that relationship as well.

EXTERNAL INFLUENCES ON THE PATIENT-DOCTOR RELATIONSHIP

In the early history of both private and government-funded health insurance, there was little concern regarding interference of the patient-doctor relationship by these organizations. They facilitated payment and allowed for

St Louis University School of Medicine, 1008 South Spring Avenue, St Louis, MO 63104, USA
* Corresponding author. Department of Surgery, 1008 South Spring Avenue, St Louis, MO 63104.
E-mail address: keith.naunheim@health.slu.edu

Thorac Surg Clin 34 (2024) 77–84
https://doi.org/10.1016/j.thorsurg.2023.08.007
1547-4127/24/© 2023 Elsevier Inc. All rights reserved.

remunerated care not only for the insured working population but also for the elderly, poor, and disabled who might not otherwise have access to health care.

However, as the health care system has evolved in the nearly 6 decades since that time, multiple influences and processes have arisen which profoundly affected not just the delivery of care but the very nature of health care itself. These include

Advanced technology: the introduction of new drugs and the increasing complexity of diagnostic and therapeutic instruments, while significantly advancing the efficacy of care, also resulted in a marked rise in the costs of care. Not incidentally, this has resulted in increasing involvement by governmental regulatory agencies as well as third-party payers who seek to hold costs down by preventing "unnecessary" care and testing. This has taken the form of prior authorizations, denials, and appeals. Such bureaucratic oversight necessitates more work on the part of physicians and their staff.

Emerging social conscience: the efforts of civil rights groups as well as the women's rights movement burgeoned since the latter half of the twentieth century and highlighted health care disparities in access to and outcomes for minorities, the poor, and women. It has become apparent that high-quality health care is not equally available to everyone, resulting in inferior outcomes and lower levels of health in certain subgroups.[2–4]

The relative decline in the physician workforce: in 1997, the Balanced Budget Act fixed the number of residency slots funded by Medicare, the pathway which produces the vast majority of physicians for the United States. Due to this residency-funding freeze, residency programs continued to train the same fixed number of doctors even though medical schools had increased their class sizes. With the usual ongoing rate of retirement, this meant the number of US-trained physicians remained relatively constant from 1997 to 2022. However, during that same 25 years, the US population grew from 272 million to 338 million, a 21% increase. The health care demands due to this increase in population were thus not matched by physician supply. The results of this mismatch are shorter visits, patient dissatisfaction, and provider burnout.

Aging population: the Medicare population carries a relatively higher disease burden than younger patients, thus requiring proportionately more health care. In the 25 years of fixed physician production noted earlier, the Medicare population grew at a rate faster than the overall population, increasing from 34 million in 1997 to 59 million in

2022, a 75% increase. This demographic phenomenon suggests there will be a growing discrepancy between the number of physicians produced and the number required for optimal care. And this trend will continue through the foreseeable future as there has been only a 2% increase in the number of funded residency slots. It has been estimated that the Medicare population will increase to 67 million by the year 2030 further increasing health care demand and threatening to overwhelm the capacity of a health care system already constrained with regard to physician and nursing workforce.[5]

Rising Medicaid population: the surge in Medicare population and costs has been more than matched by the increased population within the Medicaid system. In that same interval from 1997 to 2022 noted earlier, the Medicaid population more than doubled, increasing 265% from 32 to 85 million covered individuals.[6] While some of this increase was due to the 2010 passage of the Affordable Care Act or "Obamacare," a good deal was due to simple population growth. Medicaid-covered individuals are from a lower socioeconomic stratum and, like Medicare patients, carry a higher burden of disease than those covered by private insurance and thus require higher levels of care.

Increasing role of government as a payer: Currently, Medicare and Medicaid each comprise approximately 19% of total health care expenditure. The $829 billion 2021 Medicare costs are expected to rise to $1.8 trillion in 2031, and Medicaid costs are running on a parallel curve.[7] Once Medicare, Medicaid, TRICARE, and the Veterans Health Administration system are considered, government expenditures account for more than 50% of all health care costs. Because of increasing costs, the US government has been working tirelessly to restrain cost increases. For physicians, this took the form of the Sustainable Growth Rate (SGR) from 1997 to 2015, under which annual reimbursement cuts of 10% to 15% were proposed annually, requiring frenzied lobbying to reverse the cut every year. When the Medicare Access and CHIP Reauthorization Act abolished the SGR, it was replaced with quality-based programs such as Merit-based Incentive Program System and other value-based alternative payment models, nearly all of which failed to save significant dollars or improve quality. Physicians continue to be faced with proposed annual reimbursement cuts approximating 5% to 10% due to administrative methodology such as Pay Go and sequestration rules.

Hospital system consolidation: data from the American Hospital Association suggest that between 1998 and 2021, there were 1887 hospital mergers leading to a decline of the total number of hospitals from 8000 to 6000 nationwide.[8] The proposed advantages of these consolidations are that they will lead to coordination of care, economies of scale, and increased purchasing leverage that should both decrease consumer costs and increase the quality of health care. In fact, the literature suggests that mergers do not accomplish either goal. Due to the disappearance of competition, consumer costs rise and there is little or no evidence of improvement in quality or safety. This applies to both horizontal integration among competitors (eg, 2-hospital merger) and vertical integration up along the care delivery chain (ie, a physician group, pharmacy, hospital, and insurance company merger). While little or no quality or cost improvements result from these consolidations, profit margins virtually always rise.

The corporatization of health care: in 1930, 90% of hospital chief executive officers (CEOs) were physicians. While keeping the hospital on a profitable standing was an important goal, high-quality health care was likely the primary motivation for most managing directors and CEOs. Currently, only 5% of hospital CEOs are doctors, with the remainder having Master of Business Administration or Master of Health Administration degrees, folks who culturally look to profit as their primary goal.[9] Given the vast difference between the underlying ethos of those with a medical (health) versus a business (profit) background, it is not surprising that hospitals have evolved into major profit centers for health conglomerates. As expenditures reached into the trillions, health care became far too attractive to resist, and corporate America has taken control in the form of major health care conglomerates, Big Pharma, medical device companies, pharmacy benefit managers, private equity physician ownership, and multistate hospital chains to name a few. Bluntly speaking, physicians have lost control of health care in the United States over several decades.

The evolving trends noted earlier have led to a marked change in the one-to-one, relationship enjoyed by doctors and patients in earlier eras. In addition to these 2 participants, the examination room is now impinged upon by a large number of additional "stakeholders" including Big Pharma, medical device companies, regulatory agencies, insurance conglomerates, private equity firms, giant health care corporations, Medicare officials, Medicaid administrators, and pharmacy benefit managers. All these additional players threaten what should be a personalized, mutually beneficial doctor-patient relationship. The simple ethical duty to deliver care in a direct, one-to-one

relationship is no longer enough to get the job done. The relationship is been disrupted to the point that care cannot simply and reliably be delivered within this new construct. The professional responsibility of the physician now has to evolve to address these changes, many of which inhibit rather than enhance our ability to deliver care.

The American Medical Association (AMA) has actually recognized the evolving nature of health care and in 2001, published the "Declaration of Professional Responsibility." Alongside the usual recommendations to "respect human life," "treat the sick and injured," and "work freely with colleagues," there is a new charge.[10] It is now an expectation that the responsible physician will

Advocate for the social, economic, educational, and political changes that ameliorate suffering and contribute to human well-being.

Undertaking this type of advocacy will require the thoracic surgeons to step outside the insular clinical relationship with patients and move into the outside world to effect change.

PAST ADVOCACY BY THORACIC SURGERY

Advocacy in the specialty of thoracic surgery was spotty to nonexistent until the early to mid-1990s. At that time, serious questions had arisen concerning patient safety in the US health care system. In 2000, the National Institutes of Health publication "To Err is Human" was published and suggested that 98,000 deaths per year were due to medical mistakes.[11] The media, the public, and the government were outraged and demanded this be addressed. Fortunately, throughout this time the Society of Thoracic Surgeons (STS) had been advocating for patient safety and also had the foresight to have established the STS National Database a decade earlier. This was a first-of-its-kind clinical registry that allowed for the identification of clinical risk factors and the ability to track and report operative mortality and morbidity in detail. Institutional results were reported back to individual programs allowing for the identification and correction of any programmatic deficiencies, a process which led to safer cardiac procedures. Over time, this led to the identification and dissemination of best practices and the institution of clinical guidelines.

While this was a major step for promoting patient safety, STS leaders recognized that the database did little to answer many broader questions relevant to the appropriateness of patient care and the twenty-first century witnessed institution of several STS initiatives to address those issues.

One such issue was the widespread and uncontrolled dissemination and inappropriate usage of intracoronary stents in the management of occlusive coronary artery disease (CAD). Once stents were introduced and found to be effective for acute ischemia situations, those same stents were then widely applied to all those with CAD with little or no evidence demonstrating efficacy with regard to freedom from recurrent angina, infarction, or death. The STS felt that patient outcomes were possibly being compromised and instituted a study to investigate that fear. This required an advocacy effort to enlist the participation of 2 other organizations. The American College of Cardiology (ACC) maintained the National Cardiovascular Data Registry containing all the relevant clinical data regarding stents, and the Center for Medicare and Medicaid Services (CMS) maintained the administrative information on all stent and bypass patients covered by Medicare, allowing for long-term tracking of both survival, recurrent infarction, and repeat revascularization. This collaboration of 2 specialty organizations and a governmental regulatory agency accomplished the ASCERT trial which categorically demonstrated which subgroups of CAD were better managed surgical rather than by stent placement. Patients were now better served by practitioners who could triage them appropriately.[12]

A similar collaborative effort was instituted during the introduction of the transcatheter valve technology. After the first human implantation in 2002,[13] it was feared that, once the valve was approved by the Food and Drug Administration (FDA), there might be rapid and uncontrolled dissemination of this technology as occurred with endovascular coronary stents. This would likely result in the implantation of valves in inappropriate circumstances by less than optimally trained personnel with little or no reporting of complications and results. Once again, the STS advocated for the joint venture which would rationally control the dissemination of this technology by ensuring only trained personnel would be involved. This required active collaboration with ACC and the valve industry as well as political advocacy with the FDA and CMS. CMS agreed to make reimbursement for transcatheter valve placement, a procedure governed by Coverage with Evidence Development, meaning all valves implanted had to abide by study restrictions and each patient had to be included in and followed long-term by newly developed the Transcatheter Valve Treatment Registry. This provided for responsible, graded, and timely dissemination of the technology through the PARTNER trials which have now demonstrated efficacy in high, medium, and low-risk subpopulations.[14–16]

Other STS advocacy efforts occurred in less clinically oriented venues. In 2011, the National Lung Screening Trial demonstrated definitive survival benefit from routine low-dose computed tomography screening for lung cancer in smokers but this was not a test commonly covered by private insurers or governmental payers. The STS recognized that, without insurance coverage, most patients would not be able to afford this potentially life-saving technology and thus for several years actively lobbied for such coverage. In 2014, thanks to STS's political advocacy efforts, reimbursement for screening was mandated by the United States Preventive Services Task Force for private insurers and by CMS for Medicaid and Medicare patients.

Other issues addressed included gender discrimination and bias within training programs, an issue championed by the Women in Thoracic Surgery (WTS) organization. Historically, women were woefully underrepresented within the specialty of thoracic surgery both within the membership as well as the leadership. With 50% of medical school classes being female, the specialty workforce would soon dwindle without more effective recruiting of women. The STS began partnering with the WTS early in the twenty-first century to promote thoracic surgery as a viable career choice and promoted women within the societal leadership. While the current president elect is a woman, she will be only the second female ever elected to that position.

Within the last 5 years, the specialty recognized that the same proportional disparity seen with women surgeons was also present among other minorities including Hispanics and Black or African Americans. A 2023 presentation at the American Association for Thoracic Surgery meeting documented the progress, or lack thereof, for different minorities with regard to acceptance into cardiothoracic (CT) surgery training over the last 10 years, comparing the prior to the latter 5-year time periods (**Table 1**). Over that interval, there was a significant increase in the proportion of women in thoracic surgical training (23%–27%), but no statistically significant increase among Black/African Americans (3.3% –3.9%) or Hispanics (7.0% –7.4%). All these proportions were well below the overall proportion of women (50.5%), Hispanics (18.9%), and Blacks (13.5%) in the United States.

Recognizing these disparities both within the specialty and organization, the STS established the Workforce for Diversity, Equity, and Inclusion (DEI) to help chart a course toward rectification of these disparities within the association. In addition, the DEI workforce and STS leadership recognize that there are disparities of race and gender in

Table 1
Data depicted is from US Graduate Medical Education reports and enrollment information from the Association of American Medical Colleges from 2012 to 2022

Subgroup	2013–2017	2018–2022	P Value
Women	353/1647 (23%)	617/2311(27%)	< 0.05
Black or African American	55/1647 (3.3%)	89/2311(3.9%)	NS
Hispanic	115/1647 (7.0%)	171/2311(7.4%)	NS

Data represent the combined number of matriculants in the integrated 6 y and categorical (2–3 y) thoracic surgery training programs. Matriculant numbers are subdivided into early and late cohorts (horizontal) and into minority subgroups (vertical) including women, black or African American, and Hispanic matriculants. Numbers are absolute numbers of matriculants with percentages in parentheses. Table derived from data presented at the 2023 American Association for Thoracic Surgery meeting by Ibraheem Hazmat and submitted to the Journal for Thoracic Cardiovascular Surgery.

the delivery of CT care with regard to health care access and outcomes for minorities[2–4] and have established a scholarship to investigate its extent as well as possible methods to address the problem.

Finally, the STS has also had to utilize political advocacy to avert ongoing financial cuts which threaten practice viability and patient access. It has collaborated with most of organized medicine to try and prevent the ongoing yearly devaluation of services provided by physicians and other practitioners. While some might interpret these efforts to be emblematic of greed, in fact they represent an ongoing bid for continued financial survival.

Many stakeholders in medicine such as medical device companies and pharmaceutical manufacturers are allowed to set their own prices without government interference. Hospitals, nursing homes, and long care facilities have government-determined levels of reimbursement; however, those levels are updated on a yearly basis to account for inflation (**Fig. 1**). The physician community is the only price-controlled component of health care with absolutely no correction for inflation. To the contrary, the reimbursement has been decreasing fairly steadily for 3 decades due to frequent cuts by CMS combined with ongoing inflation. All physicians are reimbursed on the basis of relative work value units (RVUs) with each payment code valued at a fixed number of RVUs but not a fixed number of dollars. To determine payment, each RVU is multiplied by a conversion factor (CF) and that value is updated annually. **Fig. 2** demonstrates that all physicians and practitioners have sustained ongoing cuts over the past 30 years due to inflation and continued devaluation of the CF value, resulting in a 45% pay cut during that time. This has driven many practices out of business and the vast majority of general practitioners and specialists have fled to hospital employment. Patient access has and continues to be threatened by these changes.

In hopes of averting this ongoing payment devaluation, the entire house of medicine is currently advocating for the passage of HR 2474, the Strengthening Medicare for Patients and Providers Act which would mandate an annual cost inflation adjustment for medical services. Without this, more practices will fold and access may be further threatened. Again, this is a matter of financial survival for practitioners and continued access for patients.

ADVOCACY FOR THE INDIVIDUAL SURGEON

The previous section addresses some highlights of the specialty-specific advocacy programs undertaken by the STS over the past 3 decades but such organized advocacy, political or otherwise, is not the only option for involvement by individual practitioners.

There is controversy as to whether or not individual doctors have a duty to formally be involved in patient advocacy outside the clinical setting. The 2001 AMA Declaration of Professional Responsibility (see chart X) is similar to prior version of physicians' oath but adds 1 additional responsibility.

Advocate for the social, economic, educational, and political changes that ameliorate suffering and contribute to human well-being.

Some interpret that as mandatory advocacy outside the clinical setting though this is controversial.

There are a number of potential pathways for doctors who wish to undertake a worthwhile advocacy mission on behalf of their patients or society as a whole. Opportunities include addressing a broad range of social harms/inequities that exist at local, regional, and national levels. Locally, advocacy often takes the form of grass roots social efforts which could include anything from volunteering at a soup kitchen or free clinic to serving

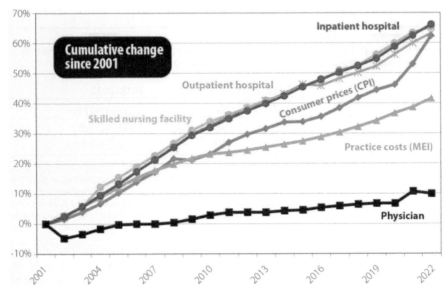

Fig. 1. Graph depicts the cumulative changes in Medicare reimbursement over 20 years using data from the Federal Register, Medicare Trustees' report, and the US Bureau of Labor Statistics. Available as open access from AMA website https://www.ama-assn.org/about/leadership/medicare-physician-payment-reform-long-overdue. (*Adapted from* Pai P, Olcoń K, Allan J, Knezevic A, Mackay M, Keevers L, Fox M and Hadley AM (2022) The SEED Wellness Model: A Workplace Approach to Address Wellbeing Needs of Healthcare Staff During Crisis and Beyond. Front. Health Serv. 2:844305. doi:10.3389/frhs.2022.844305.)

on the board of a nonprofit dealing with the homeless or those with substance abuse problems. Local advocacy can also be political in nature such as backing selected civic candidates or serving on a municipal board dealing with issues of health or public safety. On a regional level, most advocacy is political in nature. One might fundraise for a state legislator, attend a rally in the state capitol, or serve on a statewide commission dealing with issues of poverty, malnutrition, sanitation, addiction, homelessness, or any number of social ills. Advocacy on a national level is

almost always political in nature. This is because when addressing problems on a national scale, governmental involvement is required to make progress and it is the larger medical organizations that have the capability, relationships, and influence to work with the government to effect resolution. Such large organizations might represent a single specialty such as the STS or may be a larger organization representing a broader slice of the profession as whole such as the AMA or the American College of Surgeons (ACS). Political advocacy in this arena can include meetings with local or

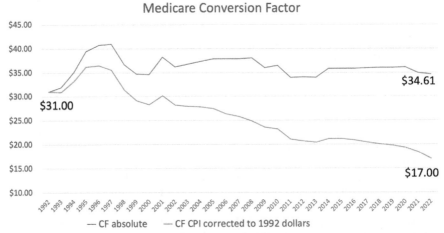

Fig. 2. Graph depicts changes over time for value of the conversion factor (CF) as determined by the year's Final Rule published by the Center for Medicare and Medicaid Services. Blue line depicts absolute value while the orange lines depict the inflation-corrected value using the Consumer Price Index calculator from the US Bureau of Labor Statistics.

national legislators, lobbying of regulatory agencies, fundraising for candidates, or writing an op-ed in favor of (or against) many issues. These may include medical issues such as access to care and medical research funding or larger social problems such as drug addiction, abortion laws, affirmative action, or gun regulation.

Much lobbying by medical societies is aimed specifically at the ongoing trends of decreasing reimbursement and increasing workloads with regard to both clinical and administrative duties. Curbing payment cuts is seen by some in the public to be simple self-interest and greed, not realizing that the cumulative effect of annual cuts has resulted in reimbursement decline in the range of 50% or greater. Such cuts have led practitioners to partially compensate by seeing more patients in less time, a practice that is frustrating and distasteful for both parties. This results not only in patient dissatisfaction but significant levels of burnout in practitioners, a trend which has led to many physicians withdrawing from clinical practice via early retirement or transitioning to a second career. In the case of thoracic surgery, those losses cannot be quickly reversed with an influx of newly trained surgeons; that is a pipeline requiring 12 years of post-baccalaureate training. Continued declines in reimbursement will lead to an inadequate workforce level with resultant access problems for patients, a problem which will likely be more acute among the poor and minority populations. Maintaining fair compensation is not a matter of greed, it's a means necessary to maintain continued access to quality medical care.

The author personally believes advocacy on behalf of patients is indeed a professional responsibility but that it can take many forms and may change in nature throughout the span of one's career depending on competing responsibilities and commitments. Major commitments might include volunteering for nonprofit services (food banks, free clinics), delivering health care abroad on a mission trip, serving on public health or safety boards on a municipal/state/national level, participating in specialty society efforts for social issues, lobbying politicians for deserving causes, or even participating in demonstrations for social causes. These are all examples of advocacy for the benefit of patients and/or society as a whole. Given the work schedules of practicing physicians, it is likely that only those most dedicated to a cause will be able to make a major commitment of time and effort. However, even those unable to undertake such a charge can and should, in the authors' opinion, consider alternate options to further benefit their patients and society.

One simple method of advocacy involvement is through a donation of time and/or money to a charitable cause benefitting society such as a human rights organization, food bank, housing assistance fund, scholarship endowment, or a religious organization with a social outreach.

Another easy way to participate in advocacy is to do so through societal membership in organizations such as the STS or ACS. Maintaining membership in such a society fosters not only the well-being of its members but also promotes the health of patients and society. Additionally, gifts may be made to the Thoracic Surgery Foundation, the charitable arm of the STS which promotes ongoing research programs as well as global outreach missions to deliver care to underserved populations abroad. The American Association for Thoracic Surgery Foundation and ACS Foundation have a similar charge. The STS Political Action Committee, as noted earlier, has effectively lobbied on behalf of our patients for many years to ensure that the needs of our patients and society as a whole are addressed. This is the major pathway for the society's political advocacy and depends on member contributions to further those goals. Participating in any or all of such societal efforts is an advocacy option easily available to all practitioners.

Some cynical doctors might feel they have no duty to be charitable or advocate outside their practice. After spending hundreds of thousands of dollars in tuition and tens of thousands of hours in training, they believe they have earned every dollar and they have. But upon reflection, most realize that fortune plays a role in all our lives and that circumstances could have been different. A random occurrence or an unforeseen, tragic event can alter the course of even the most capable people. And nearly all physicians entered this career path for altruistic reasons, taking an oath to act decisively on behalf of their patients regardless of their age, religion, race, or their ability to pay. As physicians, we are afforded by the public a level of prestige, privilege, and reward which far exceed those given to virtually all others in society. We are the lucky ones. It's not too much to expect us to give back when we can and we all should.

FINANCIAL DISCLOSURES

None.

REFERENCES

1. Hajar R. The Physician's Oath: Historical Perspectives. Heart Views 2017;18:154–9.

2. Wolf A, Alpert N, Tran BV, et al. Persistence of racial disparities in early stage lung cancer treatment. J Thorac Cardiovasc Surg 2019;157:1670–9.

3. Enumah ZO, Canner JK, Alejo D, et al. Persistent Racial and Sex Disparities in Outcomes After Coronary Artery Bypass Surgery: A Retrospective Clinical Registry Review in the Drug-eluting Stent Era. Ann Surg 2020;272(4):660–7.

4. Lamprea-Montealegre JA, Ovetuni S, Bagur R, et al. Valvular Heart Disease in Relation to Race and Ethnicity. J Am Coll Cardiol 2021;78:2493–504.

5. Gaudette E, Tysinger B, Cassil A, et al. Health and health care of Medicare beneficiaries in 2030. Forum Health Econ Pol 2015;18(2):75–96.

6. Vankar P. Total Medicaid Enrollment from 1966 to 2021. In Statista, Available at https://www.statista.com/statistics/245347/total-medicaid-enrollment-since-1966/.

7. CMS. National Health Expenditure by type of service and source of funds CY 1960-2021 In CMS Website. Available at https://www.cms.gov/research-statistics-data-and-systems/statistics-trends-and-reports/nationalhealthexpenddata.

8. Levins H. Hospital Consolidation Continues to Boost Costs, Narrow Access, and Impact Care Quality. In Penn Leonard Davis Institute of Health Economics. Available at https://ldi.upenn.edu/our-work/research-updates/hospital-consolidation-continues-to-boost-costs-narrow-access-and-impact-care-.

9. Gupta A. Physician versus non-physician CEOs: The effect of a leader's professional background on the quality of hospital management and health care. J Hosp Admin 2019;8:47–51.

10. AMA House of Delegates. AMA Declaration of Professional Responsibility. In AMA Website. Available at https://www.ama-assn.org/delivering-care/public-health/ama-declaration-professional-responsibility.

11. Institute of medicine. To Err is human: Building a safer health system. Washington, DC: The National Academies Press; 2000.

12. Weintraub WS, Sepulveda MG, Weiss JM, et al. Comparative Effectiveness of Revascularization Strategies. N Engl J Med 2012;366:1467–76.

13. Cribier A, Eltchaninoff H, Bash A, et al. Percutaneous transcatheter implantation of an aortic valve prosthesis for calcific aortic stenosis: first human case description. Circulation 2002;106:3006–8.

14. Smith CR, Leon MB, Mack MJ, et al. Transcatheter versus Surgical Aortic Valve Replacement in High-Risk patient. NEJM 2011;364:2187–98.

15. Leon MB, Smith CR, Mack MJ, et al. Transcatheter versus Surgical Aortic Valve Replacement in Intermediate-Risk patient. NEJM 2016;374:1609–20.

16. Mack MJ, Leon MB, Thourani VH, et al. Transcatheter Aortic-Valve Replacement with a Balloon-Expandable Valve in Low-Risk Patients. N Engl J Med 2019;380:1695–705.

The Mid-Career Crisis
Moving on to Your Next Job or Staying Comfortable

Ourania Preventza, MD, MBA[a,b,c,d,*]

KEYWORDS

- Mid-career • Career crisis • Career opportunities • Leadership opportunities
- Professional development • Changing careers • Definition of surgeon's mid-career

KEY POINTS

- In a surgeon's career, the mid-career has two phases: the early phase, which is approximately 10 to 15 years in practice, and the later phase, which is at 15 to 25 years.
- It is important to understand when and why one should change jobs. The playing field is usually the same, with the same issues; it is the players (ie, coworkers) that make all the difference.
- If your next job is a leadership position, you must strike a balance between promoting the brand of your new organization and supporting the people you work with.
- As a leader, you must realize that your new job is not really about you but about elevating others and using yourself as a vehicle for their success. Leadership has no boundaries.

This monograph has the following segments: defining mid-career; mid-career during the professional life of an academic and a private practice surgeon (cardiothoracic); mid-career crisis; transition to a new job and the importance of working with good, supportive people; "knowing the "when" and the "why"; the strategy for your new job; and a personal reflection.

HOW WE DEFINE "MID-CAREER"

In medicine and especially in surgery, "mid-career" is not well defined in the literature or agreed upon among professionals. After the first 10 years in practice, most physicians enter the early period of the mid-career, whereas someone who has spent less than 10 years in practice can be considered to be in their early career. However, in surgery, the physician must acquire a great deal of technical expertise that does not truly develop until years after training and repetition of technical movements and procedures, when one has considerable experience.

Any attempt to define the various portions of the surgeon's career will of course be an oversimplification because maturity, expertise, and judgment come from extensive daily practice and experience and not simply the passage of time. To my mind, a recent graduate is one within 4 to 5 years of their training, who is developing their skills and practicing what they learned during training. During the next 5 years (and up to 10–15 years), the surgeon begins to focus on an area of interest and tries to master it with time, repetition, and experience—not only performing the technical skills but also teaching them—and does research in their area of interest. Exposure to procedures, practice, mentorship, repetition, focus, and openness to criticism for continued improvement are all elements that vary among individuals and are critical for maturity. Thus, at 5 to 10 years in practice, the surgeon is still in their early career and is slowly

[a] Division of Cardiothoracic Surgery, Michael E. DeBakey Department of Surgery, Baylor College of Medicine, Houston, TX, USA; [b] Department of Cardiovascular Surgery, The Texas Heart Institute, Houston, TX, USA; [c] Department of Cardiovascular Surgery, St. Luke's Health—Baylor St Luke's Medical Center, Houston, TX, USA; [d] Division of Cardiothoracic Surgery, University of Virginia, Charlottesville, VA, USA
* Corresponding author. Division of Cardiothoracic Surgery, University of Virginia, 1215 Lee Street, Hospital Expansion, Charlottesville, VA 22908.
E-mail address: opreventza@virginia.edu

Thorac Surg Clin 34 (2024) 85–88
https://doi.org/10.1016/j.thorsurg.2023.08.012
1547-4127/24/© 2023 Elsevier Inc. All rights reserved.

developing an area of focus for their research and clinical practice. If the surgeon is in an academic environment, they are also learning how to teach and beginning to become involved in professional societies. Recognition of someone's accomplishments, a feeling of "belonging," a positive environment, and senior supervision and help are crucial elements for the individual to flourish, develop their judgment, and progress smoothly into the early period of their mid-career, meaning 10 to 15 years in practice. After 15 years, the surgeon has become confident in their skills and is able to teach them well to the next generation.

The mid-career years are very important. During this period, the surgeon is looking for new challenges, leadership opportunities, and upper-management responsibilities. It is when you are more confident and more aware of what you want to do with the rest of your career; thus, you are able to create your own opportunities to advance and develop, rather than simply waiting for opportunities to arise. These benefits come from developing a reputation as a professional and greater self-awareness. After 15 years in practice and for a span of 15–25 years, the "golden years" of the mid-career period, the surgeon has become confident in their skills, is able to teach them well to the next generation, and has the potential to shape the future of their organizations, their colleagues, and themselves.

MID-CAREER FOR ACADEMIC AND PRIVATE PRACTITIONER CARDIOTHORACIC SURGEONS

At this point in their career, surgeons in an academic environment often attain leadership roles in national professional associations and generally become more prominent in their profession. They also become more confident and begin to develop their own leadership style, making themselves more outwardly focused—on teaching and on leading. In a private practice setting, mid-career cardiothoracic surgeons begin looking for younger colleagues with new skill sets to add to their existing practice. With the continuing evolution of technology and the increasing demand for the more minimally invasive techniques, a new skill set focusing on a specific technique, or on health care management and business, is always welcome to any academic or private practice environment to cope with the demands, competition, and changing landscape of health care. This new skill set is better acquired after the early career period, when surgeons are more comfortable working on routine cases without senior supervision. The more maturity a surgeon has, the more

they can develop their new skill set in a natural way and without anxiety. Early-career sub-specialization in a particular area without mastering routine cases during the early career period can raise concerns among one's fellow surgeons about one's ability to develop the appropriate judgment, which is imperative for the rest of the surgeon's career.

MID-CAREER CRISIS

What some call the "mid-career crisis" may differ between surgeons in academia and those in private practice, and among surgeons in general. It is not exclusive to the mid-career; it can happen at any point. It is associated with a low level of motivation, an increased level of anxiety, and a drop in effectiveness. Chiefly, the mid-career crisis is about re-evaluating one's goals and perhaps one's values and needs. The one that happens after 15 years in practice is usually called the mid-career crisis.

Fatigue and crisis in a surgeon's professional life can come from constantly putting out fires, dealing with exhausting documentation, and trying to align with constant changes of rules, regulations, and metrics. At this point, you may want to seek advice from many of your colleagues and to observe them, trying to see the big picture of your own career so you can determine what steps you need to take to move it in the direction you want. The social support system continues to be extremely important. This includes family and friends, as well as coworkers. Changing to a new career in the health administration, biotech, nutrition, or wellness industry is not uncommon. Such a change can bring the excitement of pursuing a new challenge and sometimes a completely different career pathway due to the shift of one's interests, an intense need to live in the present, having flexibility, and adding a new source of meaning to one's daily life.

TRANSITIONING TO A NEW JOB: WHEN

Reasons for moving on to a new job—that is, changing your status quo—include evaluating your goals and being more aware of what you want to be and of your future career path. Moving into a new job is different from just getting a promotion or a new title at your current academic or private-practice job. One of the best ways for someone to evolve is to become "comfortable being uncomfortable."

At any time when you feel unsupported, with your efforts unrecognized, regardless of the stage of your career, you have to make an effort to change the narrative and see if you can see the environment through different lenses and discover the positive aspects of your daily professional life. If you feel that the environment is unhealthy (or even toxic) and you do not feel that you can change it, then regardless of the stage of your career, you need to move on to another job or another pathway, so you need to start planning for the transition.

It is always preferable that the transition occur at your own pace, if possible, and that you are not forced to "jump ship" before finding your next job. But even when the transition is forced, reevaluating your circumstances and being aware of your personal value are crucial. As is often said, and I completely agree with this, it is not how many times you fall down but how many times you get back up and keep going.

Lastly, moving to a new opportunity or job does not necessarily mean that you are unhappy with your current situation. It just means that you are more aware of what you want the remainder of your professional career to look like and that your current position or trajectory in your current environment does not appear to be on the pathway you want. Changes in your family life that result in you needing more flexibility or a higher salary can also lead to changing jobs or careers.

TRANSITIONING TO A NEW JOB: KNOWING THE "WHY"

When you move into a new job because you are seeking a new challenge, especially in the middle or at the end of your mid-career, you have to have situational awareness, self-awareness, and as much confidence as you can regarding what you want to achieve in the next 5 to 10 years. If you are advancing your existing career by undertaking a new job with a new and challenging leadership role, your goal could be expanding a clinical practice, building a new service line or making an existing service line more patient-centered, focusing on a specific line of research (which could include health care outcomes), or teaching the next generation "the art of surgery" and helping them move to the next level of maturity. As one of my professors used to say—and this is especially pertinent in academia and to surgeons who are dealing with trainees on a daily basis—"If you do an operation well, you can save a patient's life, but if you teach the operation well to others, you can save many lives." So, when you are attempting to choose your next job, you must decide whether the new role will make your goal attainable.

You do not want to change jobs (unless you are forced to leave your existing job) simply because the grass looks greener on the other side of the fence. Remember that it is not greener, it is just different. The playing field is usually the same, with the same administrative and clinical problems regarding surgical practice activities (academic or private), research, or teaching, whatever your focus is on. It is the players that change, and this is what makes the main difference between workplaces.

TRANSITION TO A NEW JOB AND THE IMPORTANCE OF WORKING WITH GOOD PEOPLE

What is important to realize is that in a workplace, it is the people that make the difference. The system, whether it is large, small, academic, hybrid, or private, and however clogged it may be, is created by people. Only by having the right leaders can systems and cultures improve and evolve. Visionary leaders can inspire their followers and bring about steady and positive change.

One can never underestimate the importance of working with good and nontoxic people who can support you at any point in your career and when you are reevaluating your goals or thinking about your next career move. In addition, what is suitable for one may not be suitable for others. There is a tendency for people to follow anything big and shiny, but what is shiny is not always "gold" and valuable. For example, being part of a large academic center may appear prestigious and have other apparent advantages, but if it is not a good fit for your personality, working there will not benefit your well-being. In this case, being part of a smaller system, academic or private, may be more beneficial to both your professional life and your health in the long run.

After 10 to 15 years in practice, you have developed the maturity and the insight to know that events in your professional life are not happening by serendipity; you have as much influence over them as anyone else. If you feel that you are not supported in your current job, then you have to look at yourself and see why this is happening. This is when you realize that it is not just your environment that is not supporting you; you may be affecting your environment in a way that is not helpful to you, as well. People who are happy with their situation—their salary, their environment, and the people they work with—and who feel that they are on a great career path do not leave their jobs for another job. You leave your job because you are looking for something better, more ambitious, and healthier and because your current environment is not fulfilling your native curiosity.

STRATEGIC PLANS FOR YOUR NEXT JOB

Although it is not easy to predict what the new job will look like, you usually get a sense during the interview process. The more research you do on your own regarding the new environment, the fewer surprises you are likely to encounter. Important considerations for moving to your next job include the following: When people ask you what you want to do in your next position and what your strategy will be, it is important to know what you do *not* want to do. You can only know this from your own experience, including your own mistakes and those of others you have encountered whom you do not want to imitate. You want to treat others the way you want to be treated. You want to give others the opportunities that you would have liked to have but that were never given to you. You need to understand that people do not want to work *for* you but *with* you.

And you have to have done your homework about that job beforehand to identify the opportunities and obstacles that it presents. This includes speaking with everyone you will be working with at any level. This cannot give you a complete picture of your new job, but it is essential to do. You need to see who will be happy or unhappy with you taking that position. If you are moving into a leadership position, you need to know who among the insiders at your new workplace wanted that position, too, and try to understand them and be in their shoes. When evaluating your next job, especially if it is a leadership position, you should speak to those who have left that job and those who stayed, learn about the internal conflicts, and be ready for some people to leave when you take the job. It will be up to you to decide how you will handle that, in view of your goals. You need to learn the goals of those you will be working with, look for ways they align with your own goals, and use yourself as a vehicle to facilitate the realization of their goals and yours.

If your next job is a leadership position, then you have to think about the goals of the organization you are moving into and what the organization wants you to achieve in that position. You also have to think about the people you are going to lead. You cannot achieve what the organization wants without their support. There is a balance between promoting the brand of your new organization and supporting the people you work with. Investing in human capital (the people you are going to work with) makes your vision, goals, daily professional life, and even your personal life more balanced and more pleasant, without unnecessary "drama."

PERSONAL REFLECTION

When I was asked why I personally wanted a leadership opportunity and to search for a job that would provide me that opportunity, I initially replied that it was an internal ambition to move into a higher and more challenging position, and it was that time of my career to attain that goal. But the more I thought about it, I realized that the leadership position was not about me and about putting my own stamp on the new organization. It was something that I consider larger than me. It was about the people I would lead and work with and the culture that I would be able to shape. Taking a leadership position is about creating opportunities for others, being the vehicle for people's and organizations' success, and connecting the dots to facilitate others' careers both within and outside your own organization because being a leader does not have organizational boundaries. I strongly believe that achieving these will make my own career very successful. Something that I always try to remember is that a good attitude and superior technical skill can lead to excellent performance, but a negative attitude and toxic culture, even if one has superior technical skills, can have an "infectious effect" and become detrimental to the performance of others and, in the long run, to the organization. Focusing on transparency, collaboration, and respect is imperative. Making these three things the basis of your interactions with others will help align your personal goals with those of the organization and the team.

SUMMARY

Making a professional transition is challenging at any time in a physician's career and especially during the surgeon's mid-career. This is the most important phase of one's professional life, and it is not just about being in the early phase (10–15 years) or the late phase of your mid-career in practice (15–25 years) but is about the development of experience, repetition, and judgment through extensive practice. This is when you get ready to put into practice what you have learned, decide how you want to shape your own future, and most importantly how you can help others to shape theirs. This step will help you choose your next goal and determine how you will move into the senior phase of your career and what the senior phase means for you. The more you know about what you really want to do in your next steps and about what makes you happy, the more able you will be to make the "mid-career crisis" not a crisis but a journey to a field of dreams with greater opportunities.

ACKNOWLEDGMENTS

The author acknowledges Stephen N. Palmer, PhD, ELS, for editorial support.

DISCLOSURE

The author has nothing to disclose.

Diversity in the Cardiothoracic Surgery Workforce: What I Can Do

Melanie A. Edwards, MD

KEYWORDS

- Diversity and inclusion • Mentorship • Underrepresented in medicine • Faculty development
- Implicit bias • Surgical education • Disparities • Gender discrimination

KEY POINTS

- A diverse cardiothoracic (CT) surgery workforce is important in improving health-care outcomes.
- Individual CT surgeons can work to increase workforce diversity by learning how to become upstanders and allies for women and underrepresented in medicine minorities.
- A culture of inclusion promotes fairness and equity for all members of the CT surgery community.
- Mentorship and increasing access to research opportunities are important means by which diverse CT surgery residents can be recruited.
- Success in institutional actions to promote a diverse specialty requires commitments from leadership and deployment of resources for faculty development.

INTRODUCTION

Diversity, equity, and inclusion have been subjects of more attention in recent years because the population has become more racially and ethnically diverse.[1] Yet the cardiothoracic (CT) surgery workforce has continued to lag behind in representation, especially about ethnic and racial diversity. Comparatively more strides have been made in gender diversity where women now comprise between 10% and 17% of academic CT surgical faculty.[2,3] However, this remains low when compared with the 27% of female surgical faculty or 45% female clinical faculty at academic medical centers.[3] Less progress has been made in racial and ethnic representation in CT surgery among groups who are underrepresented in medicine (URiM) relative to the proportion of that group in the general population according to the American Association of Medical Colleges definition.[4] Despite comprising 18.7% and 12.1% of the population respectively,[1] 5% of CT surgery faculty are Hispanic/Latinx, and 3% Black, comparable to proportions in surgical and clinical academic departments.[2,3] Similar mixed demographics are seen in the immediate pipeline. In CT surgery training programs, the percentage of female residents has increased to 24% but as seen with academic faculty, increases in the proportion of Hispanic/Latinx and Black residents have been modest at best. Most CT surgery residents are identified as White and Asian/Pacific Islander at 58% and 18%, respectively, with 4% Hispanic/Latinx, 3% Black, 0% American Indian, and 10% categorized as "other."[2,3] In addition, although women comprise a higher proportion of integrated (I-6) training program residents, Black residents are more represented in traditional training pathways and have the lowest match rates into I-6 programs.[2,5]

Benefits of a Diverse Workforce

It could be observed that the lack of diversity is the result of natural selection within a merit-based system. However, many of the metrics used to evaluate potential future CT surgeons are rooted in bias.[6,7] Moreover, in seeking priorities to ensure a robust CT surgery workforce, diversity and ability

Cardiovascular & Thoracic Surgery, Trinity Medical Group Ann Arbor, 5325 Elliott Drive, Suite 102, Ypsilanti, MI 48197, USA
E-mail address: melanie.edwards.md@gmail.com
Twitter: @medwards_md (M.A.E.)

Thorac Surg Clin 34 (2024) 89–97
https://doi.org/10.1016/j.thorsurg.2023.08.011
1547-4127/24/© 2023 Elsevier Inc. All rights reserved.

need not be mutually exclusive. Indeed, in this increasingly complex milieu, diverse perspectives are needed to fuel the innovation critical to the current and future success of the specialty and are linked to identity-based diversity measures such as age, gender, ethnicity, and race.[8] One need to look no further than the accomplishments of Nina Starr Brunwald and Vivien Thomas, pioneers in structural heart disease and congenital cardiac surgery, respectively.[9,10] As the number of women entering surgery has increased so have the proportions of National Institutes of Health (NIH)-funded women surgeon-scientists, although disparities remain in the funding amounts between men and women.[11] Black investigators are also less likely to receive NIH funding.[12,13] Beyond parity, the lower rate of NIH funding for Black scientists has broader implications for future health-care outcomes because they are more likely to study health-care disparities.[13]

Economic

In addition to scientific discovery, improvements in CT surgery workforce diversity have wide economic implications. The full engagement of women in the United States workforce is estimated to yield an additional US$2.1 trillion of future economic growth.[14] Specific to health care, racial and ethnic disparities in health outcomes cost the Unites States between US$420 and US$450 billion representing 2.2% of the gross domestic product (GDP) in 2018 due to excesses in premature death and medical costs as well as lost labor market productivity.[15]

Health Outcomes Improved with a Diverse Workforce

A more diverse health-care workforce can lead to improved health outcomes for underrepresented populations.[16,17] Increases in the proportion of Black primary care physicians on a county level have been associated with higher life expectancy for Black populations and a decrease in the mortality difference between Black and White populations.[18] Several factors contribute to these outcomes including increased access to care because URiM physicians are more likely to work in underserved communities and care for URiM and non–English-speaking patients.[19] Additionally, better health outcomes can be associated with improvements in the patient experience largely through better communication and trust, which can be higher with race and cultural concordance.[17] This concordance can also translate into a higher probability of patient acceptance of physician recommendations for treatment, even independent of communication style.[20]

Approach to Diversity, Equity, and Inclusion

Yet, a narrow focus on diversity in numbers alone is unlikely to succeed. Despite increases in the numbers of women entering CT surgery, the proportion of women attaining the rank of professorship in academic department remains low.[21] Although granular data for CT surgery as a subspecialty are lacking, within all surgical specialties, promotion and retention rates for racial and ethnic minorities are lower than those for White surgical faculty, especially at the assistant professor level.[22] These differences highlight the ongoing challenges faced by individuals who have scaled the barriers to entry into CT surgery only to face considerable headwinds in their efforts to advance. Sustainable progress toward a diverse workforce must address both recruitment and retention through work to ensure equity and inclusion for those underrepresented in the specialty. Inclusion and equity are interlinked in this definition by Nishii who describes an inclusive environment as one in which "individuals of all backgrounds–not just members of historically powerful identity groups–are fairly treated, valued for who they are, and included in core decision making."[23] Ideally, institutions and the CT surgery specialty as a whole would adopt a culture of inclusion as a lived and operationalized value system where complementary attitudes and actions allow individuals from diverse demographic, social, and even institutional backgrounds to thrive. Addressing this problem requires an expanded view of the CT surgery workforce, with a multipronged approach that includes attention to the future generations of CT surgeons who are now at various points in the educational journey.

Role of the Individual

Work to create a culture of inclusivity

Lack of inclusivity is one of the top contributors to a toxic work environment, and a leading reason for employee dissatisfaction and turnover.[24] The implications extend beyond the larger institutional culture within which can be found microcultures[24] where individual attitudes and actions can either promote inclusivity or contribute to workplace dysfunction either directly or through inaction. As de facto leaders in health care, irrespective of assigned titles, individual CT surgeons have tremendous influence on the microcultures in which they work.

Understand individual biases

Engaging in self-reflection is the first step to identify behaviors that run counter to an inclusive environment.[25,26] This can be uncomfortable but it is necessary to illuminate blind spots and acknowledge individual biases, which can then inform corrective actions and eventually end the status quo. In doing so, it can be helpful to avoid labeling, which may reduce the motivation to pursue honest exploration. A key element involves the exploration of implicit bias, the unconscious application of stereotypes to individuals or groups.[27] Biases are generally adaptive behaviors that facilitate more efficient cognitive functioning and are not inherently negative or positive.[28] The negative consequences occur when the effects of implicit bias create barriers to entry into CT surgery and inhibit the success of women and minorities in both training and career advancement. Devine suggests becoming aware of biases and having concern for the negative outcomes as initial actions toward bias reduction.[28] Taking the Implicit Association Test (IAT) is way to objectively measure automatic associations that can be a source of implicit bias in a variety of domains.[29] Individuals can participate in either institutional training or self-directed education on bias-reducing techniques.

Become an upstander

Core to creating a culture of inclusion is the work to address and eliminate discrimination, harassment, and bullying. Gender-based discrimination and harassment are experienced by a large proportion of female surgeons and trainees.[30] These acts range from microaggressions to sexual harassment and can be perpetrated by direct supervisors, colleagues, patients, or nursing staff.[31] In a 2020 survey, sexual harassment was reported by 81% of female CT surgeons where nearly half reported being the target of unwanted sexual attention, and 19% had been victims of sexual coercion.[30] Despite the high prevalence, direct action or reporting occurs in only a small number of cases.[30,31] When reports are filed, positive action is taken infrequently, supporting the perception of the futility of such endeavors and discouraging future reporting. Fear of reprisal and negative consequences also keep these occurrences out of formal reporting mechanisms.[31]

Microaggressions are less obvious but more insidious and are rooted in implicit bias around the right to belong in, and expected roles of women and minorities within the health-care space.[32] In instances of either gendered or racial/ethnic microaggressions, targets must often deal with the negative psychological effects and stress created by the exposure, often questioning the validity of what they have experienced.[33] More subtle microinvalidations that deny the existence of gender or race-based discrimination or constant environmental cues that a person is navigating a space not designed to include them are equally harmful.[33] Beyond the personal effects including a higher risk of burnout, patient safety and outcomes are at risk if discrimination continues unchecked.[31] The frequent silence by those who are witnesses can amplify the harm and presents an opportunity for the bystander to become an upstander by speaking up, either in the moment if appropriate, or following the incident.[34] Several interventions to combat microaggressions exist, and range from seeking understanding while providing acknowledgment and support to the targeted individual after the event or intervening in real time, to institutional policies to address misidentification and discriminatory requests.[33–35] Increased reporting of instances of harassment and discrimination is necessary step on an individual level; however, institutional change is needed to create tangible repercussions for these behaviors and safety from reprisal.[30]

Allyship and cross-cultural mentorship

The influence of allyship in the form of mentorship, support, and sponsorship to the advancement women and underrepresented minorities in CT surgery cannot be overstated.[26,36,37] Considering both the relatively small proportion of women and URiM surgeons in CT surgery overall, as well as the smaller numbers in senior academic and leadership positions, the pool of individuals from which to engage in concordant mentorship is limited.[38] There also remains scope for increased support among those in leadership, where only 58.2% of women considered their division chief or department chairs to be an ally.[37] The additional complexities of discordant mentorship should not dissuade potential mentors given the positive influence of these relationships on career advancement.[36–38] Indeed, those who would seek to be allies are encouraged to lean into exploring the gender, race, and/or ethnic differences specific to the individual mentee and should not shy away from discussions around discrimination based on gender or race.[38] Failing to acknowledge and discuss the obvious differences that influence the daily lived experiences of mentees can negatively influence career development and contribute to microinvalidations.[39] The career paths taken by mentees who are women or URiM may be different from your own based on differing goals and priorities but this does not decrease the potential value of the relationship. Education and training for mentors in best practices for mentorship and cultural competence is key ensuring success.[40,41] Seek advice from women and URiM leaders for perspective and insight into areas where potential blind spots may exist.[26] Ultimately, best practices in mentorship apply as they do in concordant relationships where clearly outlined goals and expectations will set the foundation for success.[42] Allies should also be vocal about their support for underrepresented groups and work to recruit others into efforts for mentorship and sponsorship.[43] Individual CT surgeons can lead by example through the equitable treatment of everyone who is within their sphere of influence, advocacy for those who are not in a position to advocate for themselves, and active mentorship and sponsorship across differences.

Role of Institutions

General principles

If individual actions are the building blocks for a diverse workforce in CT surgery, institutional work forms the foundation. Erkmen and colleagues outline a framework of the institutional spheres of influence through which diversity and inclusion work can be accomplished to include professional societies and academic and clinical institutions.[44] Leaders at each level must not only set the agenda for diversity, equity, and inclusion as core values but also themselves embody these principles and communicate them as priorities throughout the institution.[26,45,46] It should be recognized that values can become buried under what would seem to be competing priorities of keeping clinical and academic entities afloat. Diversity and inclusion efforts must be considered complementary and regarded as core measures of institutional success. Doing so requires setting measurable targets[47] with follow through, assessment, and accountability.[43,46,47] Adequate resources must accompany imperatives in favor of diversity, equity, and inclusion and include funding and administrative support.[43,46] Diversity leadership roles and committees should not be siloed but instead included in the operational structure and assigned equal parity to clinical, educational, and research endeavors.[46] There is a paucity of recommendations specific to CT surgery but lessons learned in other surgical and medical disciplines can be applied because these disparities are not unique to the specialty. It is also important for CT surgery divisions and departments to leverage more widely available resources because a larger influence on recruitment and retention can be created from initiatives that originate at a broader institutional level.[48] Where such resources are lacking, leaders in CT surgery divisions and departments can work with hospitals and academic centers to build the necessary infrastructure as they would for new clinical or academic programs.

Retention

General principles

Seeking to recruit surgeons and trainees from diverse demographic backgrounds without the infrastructure in place to support their success may create more long-term harm than benefit. Indeed the higher attrition from faculty ranks of URiM physicians speaks to the need for more focused attention on retention.[22,49] It could be stated that "diversity begets diversity," and this effect may be more pronounced in surgical education. In an analysis of plastic surgery faculty and trainees that included the gender of medical student deans, there was a significant 4% increase in female trainees for every 10% increase in female faculty.[50] Evaluation of the 20 largest specialties also revealed a direct correlation with a 1.45% increase in female residents for every 1% increase in female faculty.[51] A similar positive correlation was seen between applicants to residency programs and faculty from underrepresented racial and ethnic groups.[52] A multipronged approach to retaining diverse trainees and faculty is essential and includes creating a culture of inclusion, training the workforce in areas of implicit bias and microaggressions, as well as addressing issues specific to graduate medical education and faculty promotion.

Institutional culture of inclusion

The concept of institutional or organizational culture has many definitions but can be largely considered the sum of consistent behaviors, the manner in which incentives are applied and the collective beliefs, norms, and values.[53] Creating a culture of inclusion is foundational by shaping the work environment and setting expectations for how women and minorities should be treated. This includes rethinking the physical infrastructure and symbolism that represent an institution and often embodies traditional ideals of surgery and medicine such as portrait walls consisting solely of white men or media that do not bear appropriate broad representation of gender and ethnic diversity.[39] For those underrepresented in CT surgery, these symbols can be constant reminders that they do not belong.[39] The creation of facilities for nursing mothers or for religious practice is other example. A behavioral culture of inclusion entails broadening the accepted archetype of a surgeon by valuing communication and collaboration over the individualistic and strength based ideals.[54] Individual efforts to combat harassment, bullying, and microaggressions need to be bolstered by institutional action that demonstrates zero tolerance in these areas through due process, consequences that fit the violation, and protection from retaliation for those who report.[30]

Institutional strategy: plan, assess, and act

Each institution will face a different milieu of challenges in the journey to a more equitable work environment. An intentional and structured approach will ensure the appropriate interventions specific to the institutional needs. Ortmeyer and colleagues outline a comprehensive template for institutional diversity work using the acronym "GOALS" to represent goal setting, organizational change, advocacy, literacy, and sustainability.[47] The formation of dedicated committees or task forces can aid in this process. Institutional surveys to assess the presence of bias, discrimination, harassment, and bullying provide a baseline from which to measure the effects of interventions taken to address these problems[31,43,47,55] and can include use of the IAT.[29] Institution-wide training initiatives should raise awareness of bias and discrimination and equip individuals to act appropriately.[31,55] Care must be taken to choose the appropriate setting for educational initiatives that can accommodate for the potential sensitivity of some of these topics and also facilitate broad participation.[55] A mandated single instance of an hour-long department-wide training session will likely not yield the desired results. Although the effects of bias reduction interventions can be sustained, repeated training in areas of concern will be needed for substantive long-term change.[55] Postintervention assessments are important to inform the effectiveness of the educational effort with adjustments made according to the lessons learned.[55]

Support for resident education

Myers and colleagues demonstrated a significant detrimental effect on the technical performance of female trainees after the activation of stereotype threat where an individual fears confirming a perceived bias against them.[56] This may account for the findings of Stephens and colleagues where female residents reported feeling less technically prepared than men and less prepared to be independent surgeons. The findings were similar but not significant for graduating residents despite similar rates of pursuing advanced fellowship training.[57] In addition to literacy and education around bias and discrimination, improved access to mentors and sponsors and attention to work–life balance at the resident/trainee level were cited in one survey of women in CT surgery as interventions to promote a supportive environment for gender diversity.[37] There is a need for more scholarship to identify interventions to support URiM

residents in CT surgery although much of the work done to address bias on a broader institutional level can be beneficial. Early attention to leadership development, mentorship, and facilitating scholarship can equip URiM trainees with skills that could translate into future academic career success.[58] A structured 10-month program for residents at Stanford University included education and scholarship in diversity, equity and inclusion (DEI) topics and resulted in improvements in self efficacy among participants in addition to scholarly output.[58] Unfortunately, participation from surgery residents was low, and no CT surgery trainees participated in the initial cohorts.[58] In addition to the core mission of imparting clinical knowledge and operative skills, CT surgery training programs are positioned to be major drivers of increased workforce diversity.

Retaining a diverse faculty

Rates of attrition from academic medicine are significantly higher for URiM faculty who also demonstrate lower productivity with fewer publications and lower rates of promotion to professor.[22,49] In addition to the challenges of navigating implicit bias and discrimination, URiM faculty are often tasked with the additional responsibility to be a representative according to gender or race, which can lead to feelings of tokenism.[59] The practical implication of this representation and service work, or minority tax, includes additional effort expended on institutional work to further diversity that is not counted toward either promotion or compensation.[40] This also contributes to the lower numbers of women and URiM surgeons in senior academic leadership positions because diversity leadership roles, although important to improving the institutional climate, are not typically pathways to senior leadership.[40,46] A survey of URiM faculty outlined additional barriers to retention and advancement such as a lack of transparency around decision-making, promotions, and allocation of resources.[59] Respondents reported difficulty in obtaining research funding and having to manage situations where the quality of their research was questioned to a greater degree than that of non-URiM peers.[59] Overlap exists in gender-related barriers when navigating organizational culture. Additional issues for women revolve around the more frequent assignment to nontenure tracks, difficulties balancing clinical and research expectations and pay inequity.[60] Bias also exists in measures used to assess faculty performance. Female physicians receive lower evaluations from trainees when compared with male colleagues, and female physicians in specialties with low representation of women receive lower evaluation scores than women in specialties with average representation.[61] In clinical medicine, the use of patient satisfaction scores to evaluate women physicians can be similarly problematic as male physicians are scored more highly on commonly used surveys to evaluate patient experience.[62] In settings where patient experience is used as a metric to evaluate and also possibly compensate surgeons, women may inherently be at a disadvantage.

Strategies for retention of CT surgeons are linked to career advancement and include mentorship, sponsorship, faculty and leadership development, and research support. Bath and colleagues described the elements of yearlong intensive and highly structured mentorship program for URiM faculty.[40] Faculty mentors are required to undergo training on mentorship practices and cultural competency.[40] Outcomes of the program have not been reported but the intended goals are to create mentors and sponsors for URiM faculty, equip them to navigate the institutional promotions process, build bias resistance, and foster community.[40] Specific to surgery, the University of Michigan found no improvements in the academic progress of women and URiM faculty during a 10-year assessment.[41] In response, an intensive program was developed to last a 3-year period for the faculty participant.[41] Surgeon participants create an individualized career plan and work with a multidisciplinary team of mentors, supported by institution-wide mentor and mentee training, leadership development training and support as well as funding for innovation.[41]

Recruitment

As with retention, efforts to recruit a more diverse CT surgery workforce must be intentional and apply to the multiple entry points into the specialty where barriers exist for women and minorities. Similarly, institutional commitments and the engagement of leadership are foundational in these efforts. Exposure to both the clinical aspects of surgery and positive role models are key to developing interest in CT surgery. Unfortunately, there is a high prevalence of verbal discouragement expressed to medical students as revealed by a survey of Harvard medical students.[63] Although this occurs for both genders to equal degree, women may be more susceptible to concerns around the ability to balance a family with a surgical career.[63] Gonzaga and colleagues outline a process to increase diversity in training programs that includes casting a wider than usual net to identify potential candidates through outreach to organizations such as the Student National Medical Association and Latin Medical Student Association, as well as institutions that are more likely to have a high concentration of URiM students such as historically Black medical schools.[64] Efforts around retention to create an inclusive environment also bolster recruitment.[64] A multipronged approach at the University of Pennsylvania Health system resulted in nearly doubling of the proportion of URiM candidates considered, and a 3-fold increase in URiM candidates who matched, with no corresponding changes to either the rank number or average United States Medical Licensing Examination (USMLE) step 1 scores.[65]

Bias in resident selection

Identifying criteria that could reliably predict success in CT surgery training and career continues to be elusive. As schools and institutions such as the USMLE move away from ranked assessments, there may be more reliance on subjective assessments that could be influenced by unconscious bias.[6] Medical student performance evaluations collate grades and comments from student clerkships where biased wording that disadvantages URiM students can be transcribed into the final assessment summary.[6] White and Asian students are more often described in agentic terms that include characteristics such as "decisive," "assertive," "independent," and "confident." This compares to communal descriptors that are more relationship based, such as "nurturing," "agreeable," or "helpful."[6] Similar biases are seen in letters of recommendation based on gender where men are more commonly referred to in terms that conform to traditional surgical values.[66] Less obvious but perhaps more insidious is the use of "fit" when making decisions on hiring or ranking applicants. Embracing "fit" can be a way to reinforce stereotypes, excluding individuals who do not conform to preexisting ideals around who can or should become a CT surgeon.[67] Training in implicit bias and awareness of these pitfalls by program directors and review committee members are interventions that may mitigate the effects of what are often subjective assessments.[64]

Pipeline programs

So-called pipeline programs are an important component of recruitment into CT surgery and work by increasing the exposure to the specialty for groups who would otherwise have limited access. At the University of Toronto, the need to engage through virtual platforms brought about by the coronavirus disease 2019 pandemic has created opportunities for high school students to gain exposure to CT surgery when in-person shadowing was limited.[68] Such programs increase the accessibility to the specialty to a broader pool of students from URiM or socioeconomically disadvantaged backgrounds and can be expanded to other educational levels.[68] More traditional pipeline programs include extramural clinical rotations, or visiting clerkships that can not only provide URiM students with more exposure to the specialty but also provide programs with exposure to URiM candidates who they would not otherwise consider.[65] However, several barriers to participation exist including the cost of travel and lodging for students, and a lack of awareness among CT surgery program directors of these extramural rotation opportunities at their institutions leading to fewer current positions than could be made available.[69,70] Fortunately, of the programs in existence, more than 60% of integrated CT surgery programs offered funding for URiM visiting scholarships.[69] An increase in the number of clerkship positions could be an important step to broadening exposure and opportunity for URiM students, considering the low numbers represented in I-6 programs.[70] Moreover, increasing the number of funded clerkship programs would likely improve access to these opportunities.

An oft-cited barrier to diverse recruitment is a paucity of qualified candidates. While this does not obviate the need to seek out non-traditional candidates, the disparities in academic achievement present at the faculty level are also seen in at the undergraduate level where women and URiM students have fewer publications compared with male and White students.[71] URiM students applying to general surgery programs also show less research productivity compared with White and Asian applicants.[6] These patterns highlight the need for early interventions to narrow the achievement gaps with funded research programs and in-depth mentorship.

SUMMARY

Building a diverse CT surgery workforce is an undertaking that requires the involvement of every CT surgeon. Although individual work to self educate and become an ally for those underrepresented in CT surgery is critical, it is only through comprehensive, institution-wide efforts championed by leadership that real progress will be made.

DISCLOSURE

The author has nothing to disclose.

REFERENCES

1. Eric Jensen, Nicholas Jones, Megan Rabe, Beverly Pratt, Lauren Medina, Kimberly Orozco, Lindsay Spell. The Chance That Two People Chosen at Random Are of Different Race or Ethnicity Groups Has Increased Since 2010. The Chance That Two People Chosen at Random Are of Different Race or Ethnicity Groups Has Increased Since 2010. Available at: https://www.census.gov/library/stories/2021/08/2020-united-states-population-more-racially-ethnically-diverse-than-2010.html. Accessed May 24, 2023.
2. Olive JK, Mansoor S, Simpson K, et al. Demographic Landscape of Cardiothoracic Surgeons and Residents at United States Training Programs. Ann Thorac Surg 2022;114(1):108–14.
3. Ortmeyer KA, Raman V, Tiko-Okoye C, et al. Women and Minorities Underrepresented in Academic Cardiothoracic Surgery: It's Time for Next Steps. Ann Thorac Surg 2021;112(4):1349–55.
4. AAMC Definition of Under-represented in medicine.
5. Powell M, Wilder F, Obafemi O, et al. Trends in Diversity in Integrated Cardiothoracic Surgery Residencies. Ann Thorac Surg 2022;114(3):1044–8.
6. Polanco-Santana JC, Storino A, Souza-Mota L, et al. Ethnic/Racial Bias in Medical School Performance Evaluation of General Surgery Residency Applicants. J Surg Educ 2021;78(5):1524–34.
7. Teherani A, Hauer KE, Fernandez A, et al. How Small Differences in Assessed Clinical Performance Amplify to Large Differences in Grades and Awards: A Cascade With Serious Consequences for Students Underrepresented in Medicine. Acad Med 2018;93(9):1286–92.
8. Page SE. Making the Difference: Applying a Logic of Diversity. Acad Manag Perspect 2007;21(4):6–20.
9. Sabharwal N, Dev H, Smail H, et al. Nina braunwald: a female pioneer in cardiac surgery. Tex Heart Inst J 2017;44(2):96–100.
10. Brogan TV, Alfieris GM. Has the time come to rename the Blalock-Taussig shunt? Pediatr Crit Care Med 2003;4(4):450–3.
11. Krebs ED, Narahari AK, Cook-Armstrong IO, et al. The Changing Face of Academic Surgery: Overrepresentation of Women among Surgeon-Scientists with R01 Funding. J Am Coll Surg 2020;231(4):427–33.
12. Ginther DK, Schaffer WT, Schnell J, et al. Race, ethnicity, and NIH research awards. Science 2011;333(6045):1015–9.
13. Hoppe TA, Litovitz A, Willis KA, et al. Topic choice contributes to the lower rate of NIH awards to African-American/black scientists. Sci Adv 2019;5(10):eaaw7238.
14. Plank-Bazinet JL, Heggeness ML, Lund PK, et al. Women's Careers in Biomedical Sciences: Implications for the Economy, Scientific Discovery, and Women's Health. J Womens Health (Larchmt) 2017;26(5):525–9.
15. LaVeist TA, Pérez-Stable EJ, Richard P, et al. The Economic Burden of Racial, Ethnic, and Educational

Health Inequities in the US. JAMA 2023;329(19): 1682–92.

16. Gomez LE, Bernet P. Diversity improves performance and outcomes. J Natl Med Assoc 2019; 111(4):383–92.

17. LaVeist TA, Pierre G. Integrating the 3Ds–social determinants, health disparities, and health-care workforce diversity. Public Health Rep 2014;129(Suppl 2):9–14.

18. Snyder JE, Upton RD, Hassett TC, et al. Black representation in the primary care physician workforce and its association with population life expectancy and mortality rates in the US. JAMA Netw Open 2023;6(4):e236687.

19. Marrast LM, Zallman L, Woolhandler S, et al. Minority physicians' role in the care of underserved patients: diversifying the physician workforce may be key in addressing health disparities. JAMA Intern Med 2014;174(2):289–91.

20. Saha S, Shipman SA. Race-neutral versus race-conscious workforce policy to improve access to care. Health Aff 2008;27(1):234–45.

21. Ceppa DP, Antonoff MB, Tong BC, et al. 2020 Women in thoracic surgery update on the status of women in cardiothoracic surgery. Ann Thorac Surg 2022;113(3):918–25.

22. Abelson JS, Wong NZ, Symer M, et al. Racial and ethnic disparities in promotion and retention of academic surgeons. Am J Surg 2018;216(4):678–82.

23. Nishii LH. The benefits of climate for inclusion for gender-diverse groups. Acad Manag J 2013;56(6): 1754–74.

24. Sull D, Sull, Charles, Cipolli W, Brighenti C. Why Every Leader Needs to Worry About Toxic Culture. Published March 16, 2022. Available at: https://sloanreview.mit. edu/article/why-every-leader-needs-to-worry-about-toxic-culture/. Accessed April 24, 2022.

25. Price EG, Gozu A, Kern DE, et al. The role of cultural diversity climate in recruitment, promotion, and retention of faculty in academic medicine. J Gen Intern Med 2005;20(7):565–71.

26. Wood DE. How can men be good allies for women in surgery? #HeForShe. J Thorac Dis 2021;13(1): 492–501.

27. Greenwald AG, Banaji MR. Implicit Social Cognition: Attitudes, Self-Esteem, and Stereotypes.

28. Devine PG, Forscher PS, Austin AJ, et al. Long-term reduction in implicit race bias: A prejudice habit-breaking intervention. J Exp Soc Psychol 2012; 48(6):1267–78.

29. Greenwald AG, Poehlman TA, Uhlmann EL, et al. Understanding and using the implicit association Test: III. Meta-analysis of predictive validity. J Pers Soc Psychol 2009;97(1):17–41.

30. Ceppa DP, Dolejs SC, Boden N, et al. Sexual harassment and cardiothoracic surgery: #UsToo? Ann Thorac Surg 2020;109(4):1283–8.

31. McKinley SK, Wang LJ, Gartland RM, et al. "Yes, I'm the Doctor": one department's approach to assessing and addressing gender-based discrimination in the modern medical training era. Acad Med 2019; 94(11):1691–8.

32. Feaster B, McKinley-Grant L, McMichael AJ. Microaggressions in medicine. Cutis 2021;107(5): 235–7.

33. Torres MB, Salles A, Cochran A. Recognizing and reacting to microaggressions in medicine and surgery. JAMA Surgery 2019;154(9):868–72.

34. Hackworth JM, Kotagal M, Bignall ONR II, et al. Microaggressions: privileged observers' duty to act and what they can do. Pediatrics 2021;148(6). e2021052758.

35. Rubenstein J, Rahiem S, Nelapati SS, et al. Discrimination 911: a novel response framework to teach bystanders to become upstanders when facing microaggressions. Acad Med 2023;98(7):800–4.

36. Columbus AB, Lu PW, Hill SS, et al. Factors associated with the professional success of female surgical department chairs: a qualitative study. JAMA Surg 2020;155(11):1028–33.

37. Trudell AM, Frankel WC, Luc JGY, et al. Enhancing support for women in cardiothoracic surgery through allyship and targeted initiatives. Ann Thorac Surg 2022;113(5):1676–83.

38. Campbell KM, Rodríguez JE. Mentoring underrepresented minority in medicine (URMM) Students across racial, ethnic and institutional differences. J Natl Med Assoc 2018;110(5):421–3.

39. Haggins AN. To be seen, heard, and valued: strategies to promote a sense of belonging for women and underrepresented in medicine physicians. Acad Med 2020;95(10):1507–10.

40. Bath EP, Brown K, Harris C, et al. For us by us: instituting mentorship models that credit minoritized medical faculty expertise and lived experience. Front Med 2022;9:966193.

41. Newman EA, Waljee J, Dimick JB, et al. Eliminating institutional barriers to career advancement for diverse faculty in academic surgery. Ann Surg 2019;270(1):23–5.

42. Odell DD, Edwards M, Fuller S, et al. The art and science of mentorship in cardiothoracic surgery: a systematic review of the literature. Ann Thorac Surg 2022;113(4):1093–100.

43. Maurana CA, Raymond JRS, Kerschner JE, et al. The IWill MCW campaign: individual actions to advance gender equity. Acad Med 2021;96(6): 817–21.

44. Erkmen CP, Ortmeyer KA, Pelletier GJ, et al. An approach to diversity and inclusion in cardiothoracic surgery. Ann Thorac Surg 2021;111(3):747–52.

45. Peek ME, Kim KE, Johnson JK, et al. "URM candidates are encouraged to apply": a national study to identify effective strategies to enhance racial

and ethnic faculty diversity in academic departments of medicine. Acad Med 2013;88(3):405–12.

46. Vela MB, Lypson M, McDade WA. Diversity, equity,
and inclusion officer position available: proceed
with caution. J Grad Med Educ 2021;13(6):771–3.

47. Ortmeyer KA, Raman V, Tiko-Okoye CS, et al. Goals,
organizational change, advocacy, diversity literacy,
and sustainability: A checklist for diversity in cardiothoracic surgery training programs. J Thorac Cardiovasc Surg 2021;162(6):1782–7.

48. Gutierrez-Wu J, Lawrence C, Jamison S, et al. An
evaluation of programs designed to increase representation of diverse faculty at academic medical
centers. J Natl Med Assoc 2022;114(3):278–89.

49. Kaplan SE, Raj A, Carr PL, et al. Race/ethnicity and
success in academic medicine: findings from a lon-
gitudinal multi-institutional study. Acad Med 2018;
93(4):616–22.

50. Women in leadership and their influence on the
gender diversity of academic plastic surgery programs. Plast Reconstr Surg 2021;147(3):516–26.

51. Chapman CH, Hwang WT, Wang X, et al. Factors
that predict for representation of women in physician
graduate medical education. Med Educ Online
2019;24(1):1624132.

52. Nguemeni Tiako MJ, Johnson S, Muhammad M,
et al. Association between racial and ethnic diversity
in medical specialties and residency application
rates. JAMA Netw Open 2022;5(11):e2240817.

53. Watkins, Michael. What is Organizational Culture?
And Why Should We Care? Published May 15, 2013.
https://hbr.org/2013/05/what-is-organizational-
culture. Accessed May 29, 2023.

54. Bakke K, Blaker M, Miller P. Inclusion for women in
surgery involves re-envisioning the surgeon archetype: a commentary for the social consciousness
in surgical care and research series for surgery. Sur
gery 2021;170(3):981–2.

55. DiBrito SR, Lopez CM, Jones C, et al. Reducing implicit bias: association of women surgeons #he-
forshe task force best practice recommendations.
J Am Coll Surg 2019;228(3):303–9.

56. Myers SP, Dasari M, Brown JB, et al. Effects of
gender bias and stereotypes in surgical training: a
randomized clinical trial. JAMA Surg 2020;155(7):
552–60.

57. Stephens EH, Robich MP, Walters DM, et al. Gender
and cardiothoracic surgery training: specialty interests, satisfaction, and career pathways. Ann Thorac
Surg 2016;102(1):200–6.

58. Powell C, Yemane L, Brooks M, et al. Outcomes from
a novel graduate medical education leadership program in advancing diversity, equity, and inclusion.
J Grad Med Educ 2021;13(6):774–84.

59. Childs E, Yoloye K, Bhasin RM, et al. Retaining faculty from underrepresented groups in academic
medicine: results from a needs assessment. South
Med J 2023;116(2):157–61.

60. Thompson-Burdine JA, Telem DA, Waljee JF, et al.
Defining barriers and facilitators to advancement
for women in academic surgery. JAMA Netw Open
2019;2(8):e1910228.

61. Fassiotto M, Li J, Maldonado Y, et al. Female surgeons as counter stereotype: the impact of gender
perceptions on trainee evaluations of physician faculty. J Surg Educ 2018;75(5):1140–8.

62. Kuhn D, Goldberg H, Salker N, et al. Anchoring vi-
gnettes as a method to address implicit gender
bias in patient experience scores. Ann Emerg Med
2021;78(3):388–96.

63. Giantini Larsen AM, Pories S, Parangi S, et al. Barriers to pursuing a career in surgery: an institutional
survey of harvard medical school students. Ann
Surg 2021;273(6):1120–6.

64. Gonzaga AMR, Appiah-Pippim J, Onumah CM, et al.
A framework for inclusive graduate medical education recruitment strategies: meeting the ACGME
standard for a diverse and inclusive workforce.
Acad Med 2020;95(5):710–6.

65. Butler PD, Fowler JC, Meer E, et al. A blueprint for
increasing ethnic and racial diversity in U.S. residency training programs. Acad Med 2022;97(11):
1632–6.

66. Khan S, Kirubarajan A, Shamsheri T, et al. Gender bias
in reference letters for residency and academic medicine: a systematic review. Postgrad Med J 2021;
140045. https://doi.org/10.1136/postgradmedj-2021-
140045.

67. Phillips MR, Charles A. Addressing implicit bias in
the surgical residency application and interview process for underrepresented minorities. Surgery 2021;
169(6):1283–4.

68. Elfaki L, Nwakoby A, Lia H, et al. Engaging medical
students in cardiac surgery: a focus on equity, diversity, and inclusion. Curr Opin Cardiol 2023;38(2):
94–102.

69. Bernstein SL, Wei C, Gu A, et al. An analysis of underrepresented in medicine away rotation scholarships in surgical specialties. J Grad Med Educ
2022;14(5):533–41.

70. Martin AC, Godoy LA, Brown LM, et al. Cardiothoracic surgery training program director awareness
of available visiting medical student clerkships for
the underrepresented in medicine. Semin Thorac
Cardiovasc Surg 2022;34(4):1248–52.

71. Nguyen M, Chaudhry SI, Asabor E, et al. Variation in
research experiences and publications during medical school by sex and race and ethnicity. JAMA
Netw Open 2022;5(10):e2238520.

Surgical Citizenship
Engagement in Surgical Organizations

Himanshu J. Patel, MD[a],*, Stefanie L. Peters, MPA, LMSW[b], Barbara Hamilton, MD[c], Andrew C. Chang, MD[d,e]

KEYWORDS

- Cardiothoracic surgeons • Transitions • Partnerships • Transcatheter aortic valve replacement

KEY POINTS

- Surgical organizations play crucial roles in supporting cardiothoracic surgeons throughout their careers and help shape the impact of the specialty.
- In the evolution of a cardiothoracic career, each surgeon must navigate transitions successfully.
- Engagement in surgical organizations helps surgeons to form partnerships and create networks to help navigate these transitions and therefore create the changes necessary in the successful evolution of our specialty.

INTRODUCTION

It is quite simple really. Whether it is in professional situations, or personal, in academic settings or in the community, cardiothoracic surgeons are leaders. With this leadership "hat," we recognize that a fundamental role that we have is to help people through their transitions. But in doing so, we must first learn how to successfully transition ourselves.

In our opinion, the most successful careers in cardiothoracic surgery often evolve in stages, each of which requires a transition. We define three stages but emphasize that many successful surgical careers have been completed without going through all these stages. In the early stage, one establishes themselves as a competent surgeon or surgeon scientist. In the middle stage, one establishes an impact beyond themselves through various formal or informal leadership roles. In the last stage, one sets their legacy by impacting and mentoring others to become successful and thereby durably reshapes their environment. For these transitions to occur, we need to form partnerships that are supportive and if possible, symbiotic. In exploring these concepts, we look to describe the pivotal role that surgical organizations can have in providing the support we need to successfully transition across these career stages.

LEARNING ABOUT TRANSITIONS

The opening statement in a best-selling influential work encompasses the concept of transitions.[1] "It isn't the changes that will do you in; it is the transitions. They aren't the same thing. Change is situational: the move to a new site, a new CEO replaces the founder, the reorganization of the roles on the team and new technology. Transition, on the other hand, is psychological; it is a three-phase process that people go through as they internalize and

[a] Department of Cardiac Surgery, Adult Cardiac Surgery, Section of Adult Cardiac Surgery, Cardiovascular Network of West Michigan, University of Michigan Medical Center, 1500 East Medical Center Drive, Ann Arbor, MI 48109-5864, USA; [b] Department of Cardiac Surgery, Frankel Cardiovascular Center, University of Michigan Medical Center, 1500 East Medical Center Drive, Ann Arbor, MI 48109, USA; [c] Department of Cardiac Surgery, Section of Adult Cardiac Surgery, University of Michigan Medical Center, 1500 East Medical Center Drive, Ann Arbor, MI 48109, USA; [d] Department of Surgery, Section of Thoracic Surgery, University of Michigan Medical Center, 1500 East Medical Center Drive, Ann Arbor, MI 48109, USA; [e] Department of Cardiac Surgery, University of Michigan Medical Center, 1500 East Medical Center Drive, Ann Arbor, MI 48109, USA
* Corresponding author.
E-mail address: hjpatel@med.umich.edu

Thorac Surg Clin 34 (2024) 99–104
https://doi.org/10.1016/j.thorsurg.2023.09.001

come to terms with the details of the new situation that the change brings about."

We start first by understanding transitions in this theoretic framework proposed by William Bridges.[1] In this model, transitions are described as a three-phase process (**Fig. 1**). The first part is described as a period of "ending, losing and letting go." In this time, the sense of loss of a particular part of an identity shapes the period. Critical steps to ensure successful transition through this phase include linking the past with the new phase, expecting, and accepting the emotions of loss, and marking and defining what is ending and when. The second part, described as a "neutral zone," is the most difficult and uncertain, and characterized by high anxiety levels and low motivation. Yet this time is when the most creativity is required to ensure the best new path forward. Critical steps to work through this phase include strategies that not only make the phase seem like a natural evolution in the process, but those that strengthen connections and allow individuals to retain influence over the ultimate outcome. The final phase, termed "the new beginning" is the time where a sense of new purpose has been identified and marks the beginning of the end of the transition.

Successful movement through each of these phases, whether done in an organization, or within oneself, requires the right partnerships. Examples of when these phases may occur in a cardiothoracic surgical career include the crucial shifts from being a resident physician to an attending physician, or from going from a purely clinical surgical role to one that encompasses significant administrative responsibilities. As the surgeon's career evolves, colleagues, mentors, and sponsors identified through engagement in surgical organizations play increasing roles in ensuring successful transitions.

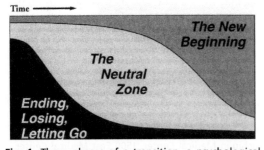

Fig. 1. Three phases of a transition, a psychological process. Note that the x-axis reflects time spent in each phase. The duration of each phase can be different for different people or organizations that go through the transitional process. Navigating this entire process successfully requires the right leadership and partnerships.

LEARNING ABOUT PARTNERSHIPS

Success in any endeavor is in large part dependent on developing partnerships. This process, termed networking, has tremendous benefits that include the following: (1) identifying mentors and sponsors; (2) creating opportunities for learning; (3) enhancing one's status within the field; (4) providing opportunities for career advancements or changes; and finally, (5) camaraderie and building long-lasting relationships.

Although networking is essential to a successful career, not all people do it well. In a recent Harvard Business Review article, Gino and colleagues described challenges to successful networking and mitigation strategies to improve this process.[2] The first step required a better understanding of oneself, namely whether one is promotion-focused ("likes to win") or prevention-focused ("hates to lose"). In an observational study, they found that the former personality type generally performed well and spontaneously networked. In contrast, the latter personality type generally avoided this process, perceiving it as inauthentic. For success in networking then, this latter personality type must view the process as an educational opportunity to make the experience a positive one. The second step to successful networking requires identifying those people who share similar goals and values. This strategy will likely aid in identifying not only colleagues but also mentors and sponsors. A third step, and likely more helpful in identifying mentors and sponsors, revolves around identifying what one brings to the table. Gino and colleagues, using a controlled experiment, suggested that those with more power and authority networked more easily and were more willing. When balanced with their wish for more gratitude and recognition, it made development of a mentoring or sponsoring relationship much easier, particularly if coupled with a knowledge of shared values. The final suggested step was to identify the higher purpose in the role of networking, such as its benefits to one's group's objectives in enhancing academic or clinical reputation.

Ibarra and Hunter described the importance of networking for aspiring leaders and followed a small cohort of managers as they emerged during the transition to leadership.[3] They described three sequential forms of networking necessary in this transition. The first form, operational networking, was required to complete tasks. This came naturally, was necessary in a managerial role, and served to coordinate people to achieve the task. Often, this form focused on networking within the organization where one worked. For cardiothoracic surgeons, this network could include nursing leaders, intensivists, or referring physicians among others. The second form, termed personal networking, evolved as aspiring leaders reoriented toward an external focus. Through networks of similar people but outside their usual circles (eg, a business manager meeting a lawyer), they closed gaps in knowledge, found people who faced similar types of challenges, and even identified mentors in a safe space. Completion of this stage led to better self-awareness and organizational understanding. The final stage, most necessary to complete the leadership transition, was termed strategic networking. In this stage, aspiring leaders built relationships to enhance their ability to learn about the broader marketplace, recruited talent, learned to work through others to enhance their influence, and eventually shaped their environment.

For cardiothoracic surgeons, operational and personal networking are crucial in building partnerships that help one move through the early and middle career stages. However, it is the last stage that we believe is most necessary to move from the middle to late stage of a cardiothoracic surgical career.

THE ROLE OF PROFESSIONAL (OR SURGICAL) ORGANIZATIONS

Professional organizations started predominantly to support their primary disciplines. As influential stewards in their specialties, these organizations help disseminate knowledge through publication of associated professional journals, raise public (and governmental) awareness of the value of their profession, set standards for professional quality, support initiatives relevant to evolution of their specialty and most importantly, support their members. An important venue for a professional organization's mission involves the societal meetings where members congregate, exchange ideas, learn about new research within their field, and most importantly, network and build relationships. In our opinion, although there is a role in hybrid meetings, there is no substitute for in person meetings to better build relationships.

Although there are several interdisciplinary societies and fields (including cardiothoracic surgery) are increasingly "cross-contaminating" with other disciplines, most professional organizations still function to advocate for one discipline. A recent publication of the National Academies describes the enormous influence that professional organizations can have in promoting the increasing role of interdisciplinary knowledge.[4] In this endeavor, several strategies are suggested. These include removing barriers to publish interdisciplinary work in society-associated journals, creating journals with other societies that promote interdisciplinary work, sponsor interdisciplinary programs and initiatives, and organize interdisciplinary society panels at annual meetings (eg, Society of Vascular Surgery at the Society of Thoracic Surgeons Session at the Annual Meeting).

The recent paradigm shift in aortic valve treatment (transcatheter aortic valve replacement [TAVR]) gives an example that highlights the impact of our national societies and their work. National society members and leaders played crucial roles in presenting new TAVR research in annual scientific meetings, published TAVR studies in our society journals, helped develop requirements for new programs and Medicare payment for TAVR, created the joint Society of Thoracic Surgeons (STS)-American College of Cardiology Transcatheter Valve Therapies registry to secure observational data, and most importantly encouraged STS members to participate actively in this new treatment paradigm with development of short courses that included learning techniques at the annual meeting of the STS.

THE BENEFITS OF ENGAGEMENT IN SURGICAL ORGANIZATIONS

The essence of surgical organizations is its people. In a nutshell, engagement in our organizations will therefore expose us to and allow us to develop relationships with other people who will provide the fundamental partnerships as we navigate through our professional and personal life. In addition, the content lifetime learning for clinical practice, including newer techniques and evolution in disease-specific understanding will often occur in societal annual meetings or associated journals. In broad categories, surgical organizations include regional and national cardiothoracic-specific surgical societies, and regional and national surgical societies, as listed in **Table 1**. Each serves a unique purpose and depending on one's career goals and potential trajectory.

Statewide surgical societies are important venues for developing regional referral patterns, disseminating local knowledge, and sharing data and quality improvement efforts. In the state of Michigan, the Michigan Society of Thoracic and Cardiovascular Surgery formed a quality collaborative initially in adult cardiac surgery and now includes general thoracic surgery to enhance the quality of care delivered across the state.[5] In its annual summer meeting, its members share local challenges to delivering care and mitigation strategies, hear talks from internationally recognized surgeons in essentially a small group session

Table 1
Examples of surgical societies of importance for cardiothoracic surgeons

Types of Society	Society Name	Special Consideration
Regional	Southern Thoracic Surgical Association	Geographic limitations/connection
	Western Thoracic Surgical Association	Geographic limitations/connection
	Eastern Cardiothoracic Surgical Society	Geographic limitations/connection
National/international	Society of Thoracic Surgeons	
	American Association for Thoracic Surgery	Academic credentials required for membership
	European Society of Cardiothoracic Surgery	
Subspecialty-specific	General Thoracic Surgery Club	
	Congenital Heart Surgeons Society	
	Heart Valve Society	
	American Society for Artificial Internal Organs	
Gender-specific	Women in Thoracic Surgery	
Non-cardiothoracic surgery	Association for Academic Surgery	Founded to develop young academic surgeons
	Society of University Surgeons	Promotes leadership in surgery
	American Surgical Association	Requires significant academic contributions
Multidisciplinary medical societies	American Heart Association	Cardiology/cardiac surgery focus
	American College of Cardiology	Cardiology/cardiac surgery focus
	American College of Chest Physicians	Pulmonary medicine/general thoracic surgeon focus
	International Association for Study of Lung Cancer	Pulmonary medicine/general thoracic surgeon focus
	International Society for Diseases of the Esophagus	Gastroenterology/general thoracic surgeon focus
Statewide societies (many exist)	Michigan Society of Thoracic and Cardiovascular Surgery (example of one)	Limited to practicing surgeons in state of Michigan

(50–100 members), and participate in an unblinded procedural data review of all adult cardiac surgical and general thoracic surgical programs. Societies like these are crucial at all levels of a career, and whether one practices in an academic or a community setting.

Regional and national surgical societies provide a larger forum in which to exchange ideas, network, and learn from leaders in their fields. Size of memberships and well-defined limited criteria based on practice location or training program location serve to enhance the camaraderie in regional meetings. Engagement in regional societies within these narrower social webs increases the ability to form networks that often lead to higher levels of engagement within national societies.

Finally, subspecialty specific or multidisciplinary societies are important venues for a more targeted delivery of information. Subspecialty-specific societies (eg, General Thoracic Surgical Club) can have novel presentation formats to enhance the education (such as "difficult case presentations"). In this narrower field, engagement by early career cardiothoracic surgeons has an easier opportunity to identify mentors and sponsors (often late career cardiothoracic surgeons). In the case of multidisciplinary societies, networks expand beyond one's primary specialty and can enhance a surgeon's presence within a new evolving multidisciplinary clinical focus. As an example, with the advent of TAVR, early career surgeons developed rapid recognition as experts in a new treatment paradigm and later career surgeons demonstrated senior leadership in its evolution. Both groups enhanced surgical presence in multidisciplinary cardiology/cardiac surgery societies disseminated collaboratively sought information and ultimately promoted a modern approach to patient care (heart team philosophy).[6]

When we view the framework of stages of evolution in a cardiothoracic surgical career, we can suggest the following. In the early stage, one should connect locally within the institution where one works and build the local network. At this stage, it is crucial to start attending annual meetings of regional as well as national societies. At these meetings, one can meet peers, learn about more senior colleagues who may develop into mentors and sponsors, and if given opportunities to do so, start volunteering in societal matters to gain exposure to people and processes. Local and regional societies can play a crucial role at this stage, particularly because they are smaller, and are better built to develop camaraderie and esprit de corps. Presentations or participating in discussions of presentations at local and regional societies in one's developing area(s) of expertise is an excellent way to initiate development of one's brand. It can link the surgeon to potential mentors or sponsors with shared clinical or academic interests.

Success with this strategy for the early stage can promote progression to the middle stage of the career. As one evolves in leadership, and network circles become wider, opportunities for societal roles and functions present themselves more frequently. Dedicated engagement at this time within surgical societies will enhance a surgeon's personal network and thereby lead to further educational and career opportunities. Memberships in workforces or active participation in presenting at meetings in one's specific subspecialty or area of expertise are examples of how to engage at this stage. A surgeon can then expect to learn more broadly about other institutions and the societies including how they function and even pursue other job opportunities in evolving leadership roles. The education one receives in these processes will likely provide additional perspective about their roles within their own organization. In addition, mentoring opportunities for the surgeon at this stage will be an important step in career and leadership development.

With help from mentors and sponsors with whom relationships are strengthened over time, one can expect progressive engagement in regional societies and enhanced involvement in national societies. Continued presentation or participation in annual meetings, leadership of workforces, organizing efforts for annual meetings including meeting sessions are all ways that one can continue engagement.

Finally, because of this collective experience, the cardiothoracic surgeon will shape the strategic networking necessary to enter the third stage of a career, where one can develop legacies that impact beyond one's career length. Although mentors and sponsors continue to be necessary, the surgeon can expect to play a pivotal role in helping shape the organizations they work in, and through enhanced regional and national societal roles, impact the specialty more broadly. At this stage, one's role as a mentor and sponsor is crucial in enhancing the mission of the professional society and helps shape the impact of the final career stage.

SUMMARY

Our surgical organizations play crucial roles in building careers of its constituent members and equally importantly define the presence that our specialty of cardiothoracic surgery has in medicine. Without engagement by its constituent members, this presence is diminished, and our specialty consequently less impactful than it can be. Therefore, as leaders in many ways, it is the responsibility of all cardiothoracic surgeons to engage in one way or another in at least one (if not more) surgical society in a meaningful way.

CLINICS CARE POINTS

- There are three sequential steps to successfully create networks that help each surgeon transition during the phases of a career.
- Transitions in contrast to changes are psychological changes and evolve in three stages.
- In order to successfully navigate transitions in a career and also successfully impact our specialty, cardiothoracic surgeons must engage within surgical organizations that represent our collective interests and goals.

DISCLOSURE

The authors have nothing to disclose.

ACKNOWLEDGMENT

J.D. Morris Collegiate Professorship, David Hamilton Fund in Cardiac Surgery, Family of Harpreet and Sangeeta Ahluwalia Fund in Cardiac Surgery.

REFERENCES

1. Bridges W, Bridges S. Managing Transitions—making the most of change. 4thedition. Boston, MA: Da Capo Press; 2016. p. 1–13. Chapter 1.

2. Gino F, Kouchaki M, Casciaro T. Learn to Love Networking. Harv Bus Rev 2016;104–7.
3. Ibarra H, Hunter ML. How Leaders Create and Use Networks. Harv Bus Rev 2007;40–7.
4. National Academy of Sciences. National Academy of Engineering, and Institute of Medicine. Facilitating Interdisciplinary Research. Washington, DC: The National Academies Press; 2005. p. 137–48. Chapter 7.
5. Johnson SH, Theurer PF, Bell GF, et al. A statewide quality collaborative for process improvement: internal mammary utilization. Ann Thorac Surg 2010; 90(4):1158–64.
6. Bavaria JE, Prager RL, Naunheim KS, et al. Surgeon involvement in transcatheter aortic valve replacement in the United States: A 2016 Society of Thoracic Surgeons Survey. Ann Thorac Surg 2017;104(3):1088–93.

The Exit Strategy
Preparing for Retirement

William A. Baumgartner, MD*

KEYWORDS

- Retirement • Social security • Medicare • Health benefits • University transition programs
- Required minimum distribution

KEY POINTS

- Planning for retirement requires diligent preparation.
- Financial planning is a key component to retirement planning.
- Selecting your health benefits is a complicated but important individual decision.
- Retirement should be a wonderful time to spend with your spouse and family.

INTRODUCTION

Retiring from any occupation is difficult, especially one that you love. The majority of cardiothoracic surgeons love what they do every day. It might be clinical care, research, education, or a combination of these missions that excite all of us daily. It has been said that if you choose a job you love, you never have to work another day in your life (Confucius). I believe this statement applies to most of us who have dedicated our career to taking care of patients with cardiovascular disease, innovating via research, and teaching the next generation of surgeons. That being said, walking away from a job you love can be very difficult. Abruptly leaving our profession can be disheartening and create a void in your life. Knowing when to retire is also not easy to figure out. Preparing for retirement requires much thought, preparation, and action.

There is no defined time line to initiate the thought process for retirement. Some people pick an age and work backwards. I had discussions with my wife, Betsy, about 2 years before I retired at the age of 72. I also made my dean aware of our plans a year in advance so he could begin thinking about succession planning.

I do not think there are many people who claim to be experts at retirement, including me. My intent in developing this article is to provide you with some factual data punctuated by my personal experience. Retirement is not generally taught, as it is personal and individualistic (**Box 1**).

It is best to have a plan, a glide path toward retirement and some concrete plans about what you intend to do once you walk away from work. I suspect several of us have not been involved in many outside activities, with work consuming much of our time. For those who have been able to balance life outside the operating room with family and hobbies, we could all learn from them.

My glide path was, in large measure, one of serendipity. In 2007, I decided to place my name in the hat to be Executive Director of the American Board of Thoracic Surgery (ABTS) and fortunately I was selected to follow Dr Bill Gay. During the first year (2008), I was an apprentice to Bill, participating in conference calls and traveling to Chicago for onsite meetings with the ABTS staff. It became clear to me that, with the additional commitments and travel, I would not be able to maintain an active clinical practice. I stepped away from the operating room and stopped being the Chief of the Division and Director of the residency program in 2009. During my tenure at the ABTS, I continued my cardiac surgery research and involvement in the dean's office as the Vice Dean for Clinical Affairs and President of the Clinical Practice Association. I loved taking care of patients and working with residents but thought I could contribute to the

The Academy at Johns Hopkins, East Baltimore Campus, Surgery
* The Academy at Johns Hopkins, 1900 East Monument Street, Baltimore, MD 21205.
E-mail address: wbaumgar@jhmi.edu

Thorac Surg Clin 34 (2024) 105–110
https://doi.org/10.1016/j.thorsurg.2023.08.008
1547-4127/24/© 2023 Elsevier Inc. All rights reserved.

Box 1
Top 5 action items for retirement

1. Develop a financial plan
2. Plan a glide path
3. Pick a social security date
4. Explore Medicare and "Gap" insurance
5. Engage a fiduciary financial planner, if needed

Board, the diplomates, candidates, and the public trust.

Retirement gives you the opportunity to do what interests you—could be a sporting activity, community volunteering—on a board or in a particular neighborhood, professional board involvement, church volunteer, spending more time with your spouse, children, and grandchildren, or become a snowbird. I wanted to try and stay involved in cardiac surgery at a national level and continue to be a member, albeit distant, of the Hopkins' Cardiac Surgery Division. Betsy and I have had the opportunity to visit with our kids and grandkids and always have our Sanibel home open for holidays and special occasions. My role as one of the 3 senior editors of the Society of Thoracic Surgery (STS) e-book has kept me abreast of our expanding field. Being a mentor to some Hopkins faculty and residents has allowed me to stay in touch with the institution I love. I am constantly trying to lower my golf handicap without much success. !☺.

If you plan to remain in the area of your clinical practice, you can ease out of practiced by first assisting your colleagues. If you are associated with an academic medical center (AMC), you can continue to teach residents and medical students, and/or participate in divisional/departmental activities such as resident interviews. If you move out of the area, as I did, you can continue to mentor and coach, using Zoom or another video-conferencing modality. Some of my colleagues have gone into industry as surgical consultants. Others have volunteered their time by working in "free clinics." There are numerous opportunities, during retirement, to stay engaged with your specialty.

I have chosen to maintain my medical license and ABTS certification—inactive status, more for emotional reasons, than practical value. Each retiring surgeon will need to decide individually what they want to continue or back out of.

As you think about retirement, it is very important that, early on, you develop a financial plan. This article will give you more details about what those plans should look like as you contemplate retirement.

Retiring across all specialties of medicine has generated significant discussion among executive leadership in AMCs, clinics, hospital boards, and society organizations. Planning for faculty and physician transitions into retirement is a critical element of organizational health, both financially and for maintenance of a physician workforce. This article is focused on retirement, but the issue of a shortage of physicians of all specialties, in the not too distant future, is a worrisome problem.

FINANCIAL PLANNING

This should be a process beginning early in your career. It is never too early to start planning for retirement. It can be as simple as maximizing your deferred contributions to 401(k) or 403(b) plans in the early years of your employment or, if available, during your residency program.[1] I have often heard, "I cannot afford to take money out of my paycheck." My response is you cannot afford not to. These are pre-tax dollars that will compound tax-free until you retire. Early in my career, we made the decision to have the maximum withholding taken out for retirement, even when finances were tight, still had loans, and had 3 children in private schools.

As you approach retirement, the primary question is whether your savings (income) will be sufficient to meet your expenses over the period of retirement. The major financial groups, like Teachers Insurance and Annuity Association of America-College Retirement Equities Fund (TIAA-CREF), Vanguard, Schwab, and Fidelity, have retirement projection instruments. I am mostly familiar with Vanguard which has a number of tools and calculators that are helpful.[2] These organizations also maintain more personalized services including one-on-one counseling with a financial advisor who offers wealth management services. The aforementioned groups' advisors are fiduciaries. When you are named a fiduciary, you are required by law to manage the person's money and property for their benefit, not yours. A dictionary definition of "fiduciary" is "involving trust, especially with regard to the relationship between a trustee and a beneficiary." Their fees are based on a percentage of assets under management, rather than on the sale of investment products.

I did not learn about fiduciary soon enough. Having lost some of our savings, we were not satisfied with our financial advisors and elected to place our retirement and personal savings in index mutual funds in Vanguard. We have a fiduciary advisor who meets with us quarterly. This strategy has given us a feeling of security.

EXPENSES

If you have been prudent and structured prior to retirement, you would have created a yearly budget and analyzed how your revenue and expenses matched up to it. In retirement, revenue is limited usually to social security (SS) and your retirement fund(s). If you are like many, you were not that structured and now need to determine what expenses will truly be. The best way of coming up with that number is to create a spreadsheet and enter each expense over the course of a year. You can then determine which expenses might be reduced or eliminated in retirement. I have continued to enter expenses each month into a spreadsheet to monitor our cash flow. If you are planning on taking vacation trips and/or visiting children and family, these expenses will need to be added to the spreadsheet. As you go forward, it gets a bit more complicated and uncertain due to inflation and other expense estimates. A financial advisor can help you "keep on track" while also assisting you in growing your portfolio.

INCOME: SOCIAL SECURITY

The Social Security Act was signed into law by President Roosevelt in 1935. It was designed to create a social insurance program to pay retired workers, age 65 or older, a continuing income after retirement. An SS tax is generally taken out of each person's paycheck while working. You are currently eligible to start collecting SS if you are 62 years of age or older or you have worked and paid SS taxes for 10 years or more. It is meant to supplement your income in retirement, not replace your salary prior to retirement. If you are able to defer benefits until age 70, this results in receiving the maximum payment over your remaining lifetime. The SS Administrations' straightforward website is www.ssa.gov/retire2. There is very useful information on this site.

I would recommend postponing taking SS benefits until you reach 70, maximizing the benefit dollars. Your spouse can qualify for SS at age 65, whether she worked or not. If your spouse has worked and is eligible to start receiving SS benefits, he or she can receive either their own earned benefits or half of your benefits, whichever is higher.

INCOME: PERSONAL SAVINGS

Structured savings, while employed, will help supplement your retirement plan funds. It requires a discipline of automatic deferrals to a personal savings account which could be in a bank, credit union, or a money market account, maintained by an investment company. You can also contribute to your own Individual Retirement Account (IRA). You are allowed to also contribute to a Roth IRA, but your designated Roth contributions and your 401(k) or 403(b) contributions cannot exceed the deferral limit, which for 2023 is $22,500.

INCOME: RETIREMENT PLANS

As mentioned earlier, contributions to a 401(k) or 403(b) plan should begin as soon as one is eligible. In many employing organizations, the hospital, group practice. or university will match or add a percentage to your contribution to the 401(k) or 403(b) plan. These funds are pre-tax dollars decrease your income tax liability during your employment and are compounded each year with no tax implications until you take the money out in retirement.

When you retire, you usually are given the option of continuing your 401(k) or 403(b) plans with your employer. It is an individual decision based on many factors. If you are savvy in regards to managing your funds, you may elect to keep the funds with your past employer and manage them yourself. Another option is to transfer them to an investment organization where they will manage your funds.

Either way you proceed, it is crucial that the money transfers from one organization to another and not through you, in order to avoid any tax implications. We chose Vanguard as our investment organization, but there are many to choose from such as Fidelity, Merrill Lynch, Schwab, and so forth. We wanted to move our personal savings and retirement funds to one organization. We pay a personal advisor a percentage of our portfolio each year to manage our funds based upon a mutually agreed upon portfolio allocation. The first couple of meetings are used to create a financial plan or roadmap which gives you a reasonable idea of how long your funds will last based upon your yearly expenses. We meet with him, by phone, quarterly for updates and assistance with specific requirements, like Required Minimum Distribution (RMD).

The RMD is the minimum amount you must withdraw from your retirement account each year. You generally have to start taking withdrawals from your IRAs and retirement plan accounts when you reach age 73. Investment organizations have RMD tables where you can calculate the percent of RMD from each of the IRAs you and your spouse have.

If you maintain employment beyond the age of 73, you are not required to take the RMD from 401(k) or 403(b) funds. However, you are required to take the RMD from personal IRAs. Once retired, you are obligated to take the RMD from your

401(k)/403(b) and personal IRAs by April 1 of the year after retirement. There is a 50% tax penalty if not withdrawn by April 1. Most people choose to have taxes withheld from their RMDs, as it is counted as ordinary income by the IRS.

One other caveat to the RMD is that when you decide you are going to retire and are at least 73 and are required to take the RMD, pick the end of the calendar year, not the fiscal year. For example, if you retire in July, you have to pay the entire RMD for that calendar year, even though you were working for only 6 months.

One result of the SECURE Act of 2022 is the 10-year rule for IRA inherited distributions. It states that all distributions must be made by the end of the 10th year following the second to die. This means heirs can no longer maintain the inherited IRAs indefinitely but must deplete the IRA within the 10 year period, following their inheritance.

HEALTH BENEFITS

One of the most confusing aspects to retirement is determining what health benefits to choose. When I applied for Medicare, I had no idea how complicated it could be. I sought help and advice from a colleague and friend at the Johns Hopkins Health Care which overlooked a variety of insurance programs. Within every market, there are consultants who can assist you in determining which insurance program best fits your needs.

The Medicare website is helpful (www.medicare.gov), but the options for supplemental coverage are multiple and complex. Let us start with the basics.

Medicare has 4 parts:

A covers hospital cost,
B covers physician services and a number of other outpatient services,
C is also known as Medicare Advantage, and
D refers to drugs

Medicare Part A

This covers hospital costs. There is a 7 months sign up period, beginning 3 months before your 65th birthday and 3 months following your birthday month. You sign up on line at www.medicare.gov. If you are still working, there is a box to check. You maintain your current health care coverage until the last day of the month you resign.

Medicare Part B

This covers physician services and a number of other outpatient services. At age 65, you can enroll in Part B. If you are still working and covered by your employer's health insurance, you qualify for a Special Enrollment Period (SEP). This period is a total of 8 months following your retirement. It is important that you enroll during the SEP, as there is a 10% (of premium) added to your monthly premium as a penalty for missing the SEP window.

The premium is deducted from your SS monthly pay or you can have it billed directly. We opted to have it deducted from our SS monthly pay. The premium is based on the last 2 years of your W-2 form. This premium covers 80% of charges.

Many retirees also obtain supplemental (Gap) insurance to cover the 20% not covered by the Part B premium. There are several carriers who administer the supplemental plans. You can compare them by going to Medicaresolutions.com. Premiums vary depending on which private insurance company you choose. Within the supplemental plan, there are choices, labeled with letters, such as "F," "G," or "N." You will need to read what each one covers to determine which one is best for you. For example, some do not cover overseas travel.

All companies are required to offer the same benefits under each plan, such as "G" but as stated above, premium prices vary, so it is important to shop the companies.

Medicare Part D

This pertains to drug coverage. Once you apply for Part B, you will be directed to apply for Part D. You can purchase Part D from a variety of insurance companies. It does not have to come from the same company you use for the Gap insurance. The type of drug plan you will choose is determined by the type of medications you are taking or are planning to take.

You will be billed separately for the Gap insurance policy and the Part D insurance policy by the companies you choose to go with.

Medicare Part C

This is known as Medicare Advantage. Simply stated, it is a form of insurance that is more inclusive of benefits. Coverage is managed by a variety of private health plans that contract with the Center for Medicare and Medicaid to provide Part A and B services. The beneficiary pays a monthly Medicare Advantage premium in addition to their Part B premium. Some Medicare Advantage programs do not charge a premium. These plans cover services not covered by standard Medicare, such as dental, hearing aids, and gym memberships. They also provide "built-in" drug coverage that is less expensive than standard Part D. The downside of Medicare Advantage plans is that there usually is a fixed panel of physicians and it is costly to go out of network. They usually do not cover you while traveling unless it is an emergency. Similarly, if you decide to live in another state for several months each year, there is only emergency coverage.

TRANSITION TO RETIREMENT PROGRAMS FOR FACULTY IN ACADEMIC MEDICAL CENTERS

With no mandatory retirement age, faculty must individually decide when it is best to retire.[3] For faculty in university settings, this often results in procrastination if no defined transition is available. As it turns out, one-third of all faculty are 55 years of age or older which is contrasted to 20% of the rest of the US workforce.[3] In a survey by TIAA-CREF, it revealed that 60% of faculty plan to continue working past age 70% and 15% state they plan to stay employed until the age of 80.[3] TIAA research suggests that the primary obstacle to retiring by faculty is due to professional identity and job satisfaction rather than monetary concerns.[3] Using these data as a stimulus, the American Council on Education recommended that academic medical centers develop strategies which will support retired faculty opportunities to be involved in learning, continue to engage in the 3 missions of service, education, and research, and maintain social connections.[3]

Based upon the American Council on Education recommendations, several Schools of Medicine have developed transition to retirement voluntary programs for eligible full-time full professors.[4] Schools have differing components to their programs ranging from eligibility and period of transition to incentive payouts at the period of transition.

Responding to data suggesting that a hurdle to overcome with retirement is loss of professional identity and a feeling of "falling off a cliff," the school of medicine at Johns Hopkins University instituted a number of thoughtful solutions. These included maintenance of the Hopkins email account and badge which allowed retired faculty to continue to receive emails via their Hopkins address and maintain access to appropriate hospital, office and laboratories, respectively.

With the encouragement and funding by the Dean of the School of Medicine, Paul Rothman, a wing of the iconic Welch Library was renovated as a permanent home of "The Academy at Johns Hopkins, East Baltimore Campus," whose retired faculty were from the School of Medicine, School of Nursing, and the Bloomberg School of Public Health.[5] It consists of spacious casual space, a conference room, computer room, and coffee bar/kitchen. It is staff by an administrator who devotes a portion of her time to the Academy. She works with the co-chairs of the Academy and the committees to develop programs and agendas, facilitates hybrid (in-person/Zoom) meetings and assists Academy members with such things as internet programs, power point presentations, and spread sheets.

To date, there are 141 members from the 3 schools, of which approximately 40% are actively engaged. The Academy meets regularly and often has an invited speaker from the University, one of the East Baltimore Schools, or Baltimore community. Three of the committees are organized to provide service to the Schools and surrounding community. They include "Advising, mentoring and Coaching," "Teaching and Precepting," and "Community Volunteering." In calendar year 2021, members of the Academy contributed 6596 total volunteer hours (2816 in advising, mentoring, and coaching; 825 in teaching and precepting; 2955 in community service).[5] Our members continue to be academically productive with 102 peer reviewed publications, 4 books, 2 chapters, and 2 patents during 2021. Three other committees are devoted to the enrichment and social engagement of the members themselves. They develop social functions and invite speakers from both within the Academy and outside of it.

The goals of the Academy are fourfold.

1. Facilitate the continued academic engagement and scholarly productivity of retired faculty from the Johns Hopkins School of Medicine, School of Nursing, and Bloomberg School of Nursing
2. Connect retired faculty with opportunities for service to Johns Hopkins University, the Baltimore community, and society at large
3. Offer retired faculty diverse opportunities for continued learning
4. Help retired faculty maintain their social and professional connections within Johns Hopkins

Although it is still early in its establishment (the wing in the Welch Library was dedicated in October, 2018), it is well-regarded by its members and the students, faculty, and surrounding community who have benefitted from the members' wisdom, expertise, and time.

ESTABLISHING STATE RESIDENCE

Although this might not pertain to most people retiring, I thought it would be important to include because there are specific rules that you need to follow if you switch your primary residence. For us, it was an easy decision. We had been going to Sanibel for over 50 years and had acquired Betsy's family home. We love the island, which is currently recovering from the devastating effects of hurricane Ian. Since we were going to make Sanibel our primary or principal residence, we contacted an attorney on Sanibel to understand what conditions needed to be met and what rules to follow. Interesting, there is no definition of principal residence in the tax code. There is a "183-day" IRS rule which applies to states that have a state income tax. This means that, if you plan to spend time during retirement in the state you practiced medicine in, you have to spend at least 183 days outside that particular state to avoid paying state income tax.

There is an obvious benefit of living in a state without state income taxes or estate taxes. Some states do not tax retirement distributions and others do not tax SS benefits.

Establishing primary residence requires having a number of documents issued in the state of residence. These include, but are not limited to, a driver's license, voter registration, primary mailing address, utility bills, and car license. These, along with the 183-day rule, are important to document your principal residence.

SUMMARY

What I have enjoyed most in my retirement of 4 years has been spending more time with my wife, children, and grandchildren, while living on Sanibel island in Southwest Florida. I have ample time to run, exercise, bike, and play golf, all of which Betsy and I often do together. Most of what I have read about "getting older" focuses on staying active, both physically and mentally to stay healthy.

I have been fortunate to remain connected to Johns Hopkins through the Academy and the Division of Cardiac Surgery. I have time to mentor and continue as one of the senior editors of the STS e-book. I also started a family chronicle that includes memorabilia which is meant for our kids and grandkids. I am often asked if I miss work? Although I loved each one of my roles at Johns Hopkins over the 37 years, I miss most my interactions with my friends and colleagues at the hospital and health system.

I think if you adequately prepare and create a type of glide path for retirement, you and your spouse will greatly enjoy retirement years!

DISCLOSURE

The author has nothing to disclose.

REFERENCES

1. Quinn JB, editor. Smart and simple financial strategies for Busy people. New York: Simon & Schuster; 2006. p. 27.
2. Vanguard Tools Repository. In Vanguard. Available at: https://investor.vanguard.com/tools-calculators/overview.
3. Baumgartner W, Ziminski C, VanBeek J, et al. Everybody wins when Retiring Faculty of Health Professions Schools are Supported. Acad Med 2021; 96(10):1375–6.
4. Senior Faculty Retirement Resources Overview. In: Johns Hopkins School of Medicine: The Office of Faculty Development. Available at: https://www.hopkinsmedicine.org/fac_development/sr-faculty-retirement-resources/index.html#:~:text=Senior%20Faculty%20Transition%20Programs%20The%20Johns%20Hopkins%20University,and%20transparent%20pathways%20to%20retirement%20for%20full-time%20faculty. Accessed February 26, 2023.
5. The Academy at Johns Hopkins, East Baltimore Campus. In Johns Hopkins School of Medicine. Available at: https://www.hopkinsmedicine.org/the-academy/. Accessed February 26, 2023.

Moving?

Make sure your subscription moves with you!

To notify us of your new address, find your **Clinics Account Number** (located on your mailing label above your name), and contact customer service at:

Email: journalscustomerservice-usa@elsevier.com

800-654-2452 (subscribers in the U.S. & Canada)
314-447-8871 (subscribers outside of the U.S. & Canada)

Fax number: 314-447-8029

Elsevier Health Sciences Division
Subscription Customer Service
3251 Riverport Lane
Maryland Heights, MO 63043

ELSEVIER